CONQUERING MENOPAUSE:

MASTER YOUR SYMPTOMS TO REGAIN YOUR VITALITY
AND FEEL LIKE YOURSELF AGAIN

SAMARRA JAMES

TABLE OF CONTENTS

INTRODUCTION

If life is a canvas, then menopause has to be the brushstroke—bold and unpredictable, with the ability to change a woman's life forever.

Understanding that you may have entered or are a few years away from menopause is a tough yet certain realization all women have to go through at a certain time in their lives.

Simply put, menopause is a time in a woman's life when her monthly periods stop making an appearance after 12 months of perimenopause. Although the symptoms of menopause can last more than 10 years, it's a phenomenal transition from having childbearing years to non-childbearing years.

It's a time of extreme hormonal changes that commonly occur either in the late 30s or 40s or when a woman hits her early 50s. It's marked as a change not only because of the biological reasons but also the hormonal, physical, and emotional adjustments that come along with it.

FACTS ABOUT MENOPAUSE YOU SHOULD KNOW

If you find yourself getting extremely cranky, feeling frustrated, or having a mental breakdown accompanied by irregular periods, you may have entered the perimenopause phase. It is during perimenopause that your ovaries start to shut down because of a gradual loss of estrogen.

Menopause is identified by the surge of physical symptoms that follow it. These symptoms can include:

- hot flashes and night sweats
- disturbed patterns of sleep
- fluctuating mood changes
- vaginal dryness
- sexual problems
- cognitive and urinary tract issues

Once you go an entire year without periods, that's when you have officially entered menopause.

Nonetheless, it's not shocking when we say that many women are not prepared for such a monumental shift in their lives. Some studies show that women above the age of 40 have limited to no knowledge about this imperative topic (Munn, C. et al., 2022).

MENOPAUSAL STRUGGLES

Many women regard menopause as a glorifying period where they are finally free of periods and do not have to go through the vigorous pregnancy stage, but there are some long-term complications of menopause as well. These problems can include osteoporosis, cardiovascular diseases, metabolic changes, and quite a few more.

Would you believe me if I told you that so many women feel the same way you might be feeling because of these changes in your body?

As a society, we don't often disregard these problems. We expect women to do everything magically and not show even the slightest hint of a frown on their faces. Many women don't view menopause as a biological shift but a daily confrontation that they have to face while hiding themselves in the dark corners of their rooms.

Sudden hot flashes may leave a seemingly normal and calm moment burning like wildfire or may drown your sanctuary of rest in night sweats. Tears may roll down your cheeks, or the simplest of tasks may morph into a never-ending battle.

Navigating this time of your life is nothing less than a puzzling labyrinth where the struggle of achieving that core balance is accompanied by challenges of fatigue, mood swings, and hormonal changes.

Yet, despite all of this, we women pick ourselves up each and every day and face the unknown with courage, resiliency, and grace. This transformative struggle is not a mere achievement but proof of strength and bravery.

In addition, you may also feel unsure of what your life will look like in the years of being a postmenopausal woman. This is where this book comes in to save the day!

FEELING LOST? DON'T WORRY, YOU'RE IN SAFE HANDS!

Conquering menopause is not about fighting your symptoms. Instead, it is about embracing that rhythm of change.

This book will gently take your hand and guide you through all the changes you'll face. It will be a safe space for you to confide your fears. You will be taught how to deal with your symptoms, how to prioritize yourself in this journey, and how to feel comfortable in your skin.

Don't think of this book as only words filled with information. Instead think of this book as your ally that will offer you insights, strategies, and a dash of humor to navigate this unique phase of your life.

I want you to picture this book as a road map to victory, a guide that will help you through that foggy terrain of your night sweats and the dangerous-feeling roller coaster of your emotions.

You can walk this path knowing that we are in this together. We'll also be peeling back the layers of myths and misconceptions surrounding menopause.

Let's uncover the power behind every symptom. From the laughter that accompanies the hot flashes to the wisdom etched in the sleepless nights, every error becomes the brushstroke in the art of your resilience.

WILL THIS BOOK ALIGN WITH YOUR INTERESTS AND OBJECTIVES?

Absolutely! Dealing with menopause is not an easy task. Without a handful of good advice, you may feel lost and not know where to look for answers.

This comprehensive book will allow you to gather useful information that will not only make you feel confident while facing menopause but will also comfort you in a way that feels like a hug.

As we delve into conquering menopause, remember that you are not alone in this journey. In addition to this book being a virtual portal of knowledge you can source to empower yourself, it will serve as a reminder that you possess the power to overcome the challenges menopause will throw at you.

Buckle up for an expedition of self-discovery, a journey where your symptoms will turn into stepping stones and where getting the best of menopause is not just a mere possibility but an inevitability. The adventure begins here!

Before you get into Chapter 1, I want you to recite these affirmations out loud:

- I love myself just the way I am.
- I am beautiful regardless of my shape and size.
- I am powerful beyond measure.
- I am happy where I am in life.
- I'm confident in my skin.
- I respect my body for all it does for me on the daily.
- I accept myself with all the flaws that make me; me.
- I approach menopause with an open mind and heart.
- I believe in myself and my energy.
- I am grateful for all the experiences life has given me; the good ones and the bad ones, too.

1

GRACEFUL AGING

So many women I've talked to see menopause as an ending. But I've discovered this is your moment to reinvent yourself after years of focusing on the needs of everyone else. It's your opportunity to get clear about what matters to you and then to pursue that with all of your energy, time, and talent.

— OPRAH WINFREY

As a woman journeys through various changes in her life, few of them are as transformative as menopause. Graceful aging in menopause means navigating the experience with a positive mindset, embracing the changes, and opting for a healthier lifestyle during this transition.

In this chapter, we will delve into the intricacies of this process and how it affects women physically, mentally, and socially.

UNDERSTANDING MENOPAUSE BASICS

Menopause is diagnosed in a woman's life when she spends a year without her monthly periods making an appearance. This stage typically occurs around the late 40s and early 50s.

At this point, a woman's ovaries stop producing eggs for fertilization. However, it's not like a woman directly jumps to this stage. Before menopause becomes a permanent shift in her life, she goes through something called perimenopause. So, to comprehensively understand menopause, we must know its stages, listed below:

Stage 1: Perimenopause

Perimenopause is the transition to menopause. It marks the end of a woman's reproductive years and is also called the menopausal transition. Because all of us women are unique in our shapes, ways, and designs, there isn't a specific age when the body starts going through perimenopause symptoms.

On average, this stage lasts for seven years, but it can be longer or shorter. During this time, the body has less estrogen and progesterone, the hormones responsible for regulating the monthly cycle (Fernandes, 2023).

A shift in these hormones can lead to experiencing symptoms you have never had before. For instance, you may notice that your periods become irregular and you suddenly get hot flashes.

Since it can be a frustrating and challenging time, it's important to take care of yourself. Ensure that you are eating healthy, working out, and engaging with friends and family you can lean on for support and encouragement.

During the transition from perimenopause to menopause, women get irregular periods, and at times, the flow and days are heavier and longer and vice versa.

Stage 2: Menopause

Menopause can affect you emotionally and socially as well. You may feel anxious, insecure, and even depressed as the physical changes in your body occur. The following can be symptoms you experience during and following the menopausal transition, which can vary:

- **Irregular periods:** As your ovulation becomes unpredictable, you will find that your periods are either shorter or longer, lighter or heavier. You may even skip your periods.
- **Night sweats and hot flashes:** A hot flash is described as this sudden wave of heat that takes over, and it is usually accompanied by heavy sweating. Hot flashes most often take place during nighttime and can vary in intensity and duration. They can even cause disturbances in your sleep, and you may find yourself lying awake in bed at 3 a.m. on a Tuesday.
- **Vaginal dryness:** Decreased estrogen levels can lead to your vagina feeling dry. The loss in elasticity and lubrication may make you feel unwanted or self-conscious during intimacy.
- **Mood swings:** Due to the hormonal changes, you may find yourself going through a mix of emotions. Waves of sadness and depression may come across on a seemingly normal day—just remember that it's okay to feel that way.
- **Weight gain and fatigue:** During menopause, women often encounter the phenomenon known as "menopot" or

"menopause spread," which involves an increase in weight, typically concentrated in the abdominal area (Levine & Smythe, n.d.). Some women also go through fatigue and experience low energy levels in general.

- **Fertility window:** As long as you're having periods, even if they are irregular, there is a chance to conceive and get pregnant. Subsequently, if you stop having them, you can't get pregnant, and your time as a fertile woman has come to an end.

Stage 3: Postmenopause

Once you have been without a period for a year, you are considered to be postmenopausal. This is also when the hot flashes and other symptoms get milder or go away. Postmenopause is a new stage in life that should be embraced.

Unfortunately, upon entering this stage, you're now prone to some serious health risks. It's important to know when you have entered this stage because postmenopausal bleeding is dangerous, and you should check with a doctor immediately if you experience it.

Here are some common health issues you may face during this stage:

- **Cardiovascular issues:** The hormone estrogen is vital for a woman's health even outside of her menstrual cycle. It has a positive effect on the lining of the heart arteries, as it helps in regulating blood flow. Because of a decrease in estrogen, it is noted that after menopause, women are at an increased risk of heart disease (*Postmenopause: Signs, Symptoms, & Treatments*, n.d.).
- **Osteoporosis:** Since there is a direct relationship between lack of estrogen after menopause, women can be

susceptible to osteoporosis. Osteoporosis is a condition that makes the bones brittle and weak.

- **Urinary problems:** When estrogen levels drop, the lining of the urethra may become thinner. Additionally, as women age or go through vaginal childbirth, the muscles around the urethra may weaken. This can raise the chances of experiencing bladder leakage.

If any of these problems or any additional concerning issue arises, consult your healthcare provider immediately and get yourself checked.

DEBUNKING COMMON MENOPAUSE MISCONCEPTIONS

It's next to impossible for something as common as menopause to not have a bunch of misconceptions surrounding it. So, let's debunk some of the most popular myths you may have come across.

Myth 1: Get used to the symptoms. You don't need to see a doctor.

Even if your symptoms are mild to moderate but are making you uncomfortable, affecting your personal relationships, or pushing you toward depression, consult with a doctor as soon as you can.

You shouldn't hesitate to speak up about your emotions or when considering treatment. Don't let anyone guilt trip you into thinking that looking after yourself is selfish. Medical treatment for your symptoms is available. Book an appointment and see a healthcare provider now.

Myth 2: Once you enter menopause, you're an old woman. Everything about life is going to be a nuisance now.

Menopause doesn't mean that you are a haggard woman no one wants to be around. In fact, it's a time that indicates a special change in your life and opens the doors for new opportunities.

Menopause can be one of the most liberating times for women. You no longer have to worry about contraceptives or period pains! Women can emerge happy and powerful and should celebrate the freedom the new stage brings.

Myth 3: Stay away from hormone therapy. It's unsafe.

For some women, hormonal therapy, accompanied by prescription pills and patches, can be safe and effective. In some cases, it can alleviate symptoms completely.

According to the North American Menopause Society, even though using hormones can increase your risk of breast cancer and cardiovascular diseases, research indicates that for healthy women under 60 experiencing significant hot flashes, the advantages of hormone therapy may be greater than the potential risks.

The aim is to use the smallest amount of hormone therapy needed to relieve symptoms for the shortest duration required. Also, if a woman has a uterus, it's necessary to combine estrogen with progestogen (*Don't Sweat It: Busting Six Menopause Myths*, 2022).

WHICH STAGE AM I IN?

At times, it can be hard to decipher which stage of menopause you are going through. Although menopause is confirmed when a woman has gone without a menstrual period for 12 months in a row, before reaching it during the perimenopause phase, menstrual cycles can become irregular. This means that the length of the menstrual cycle and associated symptoms may change during the period leading up to menopause and make it hard to know what stage you're in.

Aside from the symptoms of all three stages we've discussed, you can also track your period cycle. You can use any of the following methods to track your period adeptly.

- **Using a calendar:** You can keep a menstrual calendar where you can physically mark the dates or keep a period-tracking app such as Flo, Clue, or Glow. Make notes of any changes in your symptoms that occur from the start to the finish. I personally like to do it in an app, and it's so helpful.
- **Noting your cycle length:** Keep an eye on the length of your cycle if you don't want a calendar. During perimenopause, menstrual cycles may either lengthen or shorten from the usual duration, and there can be variations in cycle length from one menstrual period to the next.
- **Tracking menstrual flow:** The flow of your menstrual cycles can determine a lot about your symptoms. If you are having a heavy flow, you may be in the early stages of perimenopause. If you are having a lighter flow, you may be in the last stages of perimenopause, also called borderline menopause stages.
- **Testing hormones:** If you don't want to use calendars or keep an eye on your cycle length, then opt for hormone tracking. Some women choose to track their hormones through home hormone testing kits. These kits can measure levels of your hormones such as estrogen and

progesterone in your saliva or urine, providing awareness of your hormonal fluctuations. You can purchase them online or through a medical store.

- **Consulting with a healthcare provider:** If you try all of the available options but still don't feel satisfied, then that's your cue to consult a healthcare provider. They can help you track your menstrual patterns and give you further guidance as well.

EMBRACING CHANGE AND AGING POSITIVELY

Since menopause can come with severe symptoms such as hot flashes, vaginal dryness, night sweats, and mood swings, it's not something women often look forward to.

Although it marks the end of your fertile years, it's not the end of the road. In fact, research claims that the average life expectancy of women in the United States is 81 years (*It's Not All Bad: 5 Positive Parts of Menopause*, n.d.). That means you have nearly half your life left to live!

So, instead of sulking about how menopause is the end of good years in your life, let's look at some of the positives that will make you feel better about the process:

- **No more periods:** One of the main perks enjoyed by postmenopausal women overall is the freedom from periods. Imagine not having to worry about pads or tampons, leakage, and, most importantly, those dreaded mood swings that irritate your attitude right before an important event. In fact, women who are anemic and suffer from heavy period flow often find their energy revitalized upon being done with periods.

- **No risk of pregnancy:** Women who enjoy sexual intercourse can finally do so without even thinking of a possible pregnancy. By the time menopause is a permanent thing, your body stops ovulation. This means you no longer have to use contraceptives—or deal with their unpleasant side effects, depending on which method you used to use.
- **Relief from menstrual symptoms:** Some women suffer from menstrual migraines, which include headaches, sweats or chills, and vomiting. Research recorded that about 60% of the women who have menstrual migraines have found a connection between migraines and menstruation (Upham & Smythe, 2023). Although your hormonal changes are responsible for your mood swings, fluctuating hormonal changes can make them worse. But by the time menopause rolls around, your estrogen and progesterone levels decline, and those menstrual symptoms stop, too. You can also kiss your premenstrual syndrome (PMS) goodbye forever—as well as the symptoms such as bloating, cramps, and headaches that often come with it.
- **Disappearing body hair:** If you are someone who is always stressed about your wax appointments and shaving days, you'll be more than happy to know that menopause gets rid of a lot of unwanted hair for you. Those declining hormones not only eliminate your period symptoms, but they can also make your hair grow slower or not at all.

Moments of Menopause Mastery

Now, let's look at some tales of women who went through menopause and came out stronger than ever.

Lilly's Revamp

After years of dedicating her services to her career and family, Lilly entered menopause. She was immediately hit with uncertainty about her body and struggled with fatigue on the daily.

That was until she decided to take care of herself. By joining the reader's club, just like she did in her high school years, Lilly did something she loved and had always wanted to do but never had the time for.

She found her passion and creativity again. After the youthful years of her life, she felt herself come to life once again in her senior years. She saw a huge decrease in her anxiety and depression. Two months into it, she realized it had been a long time since she took an antidepressant.

Rose's Path to Empowerment

Rose, a successful business owner, faced her menopause with grace and eloquence. Instead of letting the process weigh her down, she improvised and started taking care of herself through yoga and meditation.

After a few years, she decided to create her own menopause support group and invited women from her community and business to join hands and make menopause a journey of collective strength and empowerment.

Tasha's Fitness Evolution

Upon hitting her early 50s, Tasha decided to direct herself to fitness when her menopause made an appearance.

She was concerned about being at risk of osteoporosis, so she started a fitness regimen that focused on cardiovascular exercises and strength training. She found herself in better shape, and she also realized that her mood swings had significantly improved.

PSYCHOLOGICAL EFFECTS OF MENOPAUSE

When entering this stage, not a lot of women expect their mental health to be affected due to menopause. However, due to the imbalance of hormones, it is most likely that your mood will be affected as well, often including feelings of depression, anxiety, and stress. Some symptoms of menopause may also include forgetfulness, irritability, low self-esteem, poor concentration, and loss of confidence.

Menopause can cause an increased risk of depression. So, it's important to realize that the mental symptoms can just be as severe as the physical ones. Don't hesitate to consult with your doctor if you are working on improving your emotional well-being but think you might need some professional advice (*Menopause and Your Mental Wellbeing*, 2022).

How to Build a Positive Mindset

As you enter menopause, maintaining a positive mindset can be emotionally draining. However, you can adopt the following behaviors and tailor them to you. Remember, no one can save you but yourself:

- **Identify areas to change:** You cannot become a better version of yourself if you don't point out your areas of change. You can start by self-reflecting, paying attention to your emotions, and filtering your reactions. Notice recurring negative patterns and try to identify what triggers you.

- **Check yourself:** To become mindful, incorporate the habit of regular self-checks. Don't beat yourself up when talking to yourself internally. Ensure that the language you use lifts you and inspires you to do better.
- **Be open to humor:** You may have heard the saying, "Laughter is the best medicine." Indeed, laughing makes you feel better. Keep yourself open to little jokes here and there. Life's tough already, and finding small ways to keep yourself happy surely goes a long way.
- **Follow a healthy lifestyle:** Most of us don't realize how much of a blessing our health is until it starts slipping out of our hands. Maintaining a healthy lifestyle is integral when it comes to wanting a positive mindset, too. Take part in physical activities that keep you energized. You have a miraculous body, and giving it the proper nutrition to maintain your health will give you the tools to thrive.
- **Surround yourself with positive people:** We are defined by the company we keep. If you surround yourself with people who see the better in you even during your worst day that will teach you to be kinder to yourself. If you want a positive mindset, surround yourself with people who support and inspire you.
- **Practice positive self-talk:** Embrace a mindset that views the negatives as temporary and valuable lessons. Focus on the small achievements of your journey, not simply the destination. Say positive affirmations to yourself daily. Over time, this habit will reshape not only your thoughts but how you choose to act upon them, too.

The Power of Intention

Going into menopause is not the time to fear. Open your arms and mind and embrace the change. Set an intention to view menopause as a time when you can begin to explore new possibilities. Pick up a new hobby, start exercising, or do something that makes you *you*. Don't restrict yourself by thinking this process will end the happy days of your life.

If you haven't been on the right track in your life, treat menopause as your turning point and determine to make things better for yourself in the future. Redefine your goals, purpose, and relationships. Do whatever it takes to not lose yourself by being overwhelmed.

HORMONAL CHANGES AND THEIR EFFECTS

Beginning in the perimenopause stage, the level of hormones produced by the ovaries is constantly fluctuating. This happens mainly to the female hormone known as estrogen. Estrogen is responsible for a lot of different functions in your body. From keeping your vagina moisturized to maintaining the level of blood supplied—it's all handled by estrogen (*Changes in Hormone Levels*, n.d.).

When your estrogen levels drop rapidly and become quite low, you start to experience hot flashes and night sweats, which happen to be two of the most classic symptoms of menopause. Because of this, you may find your energy levels drained. Not only that, but reduced levels of estrogen and progesterone (from the perimenopause level) can cause vaginal dryness that can affect your sexual activity.

Long-Term Health Implications of Menopause

As discussed in the postmenopause stage, some health implications occur in women as well. Let's delve into them in more detail:

- **Postmenopausal osteoporosis and bone health:** After the age of 30, women start to lose the bone tissue responsible for maintaining their rigidity due to the loss of estrogen, as it sustains bone density. So, you are at risk of breaking your bones more easily at this stage. Osteoporosis develops when your body loses too much bone, doesn't make enough bone, or both. However, osteopenia means that you happen to have low bone density, but it's not as severe as osteoporosis (DePolo, n.d.).
- **Cardiovascular health:** Estrogen protects you from cardiovascular issues such as stroke and heart attacks. Without it around, you become prone to these conditions. Being less active and not taking care of what you eat can lead to high blood pressure and high cholesterol. If you happen to smoke or don't have a healthier lifestyle, start making those changes to ensure better health.
- **Urinary and vaginal changes:** When estrogen levels decrease during menopause, it can cause discomfort during urination, more frequent trips to the bathroom, and difficulty holding urine (incontinence). Lower estrogen can also bring about changes in the vagina, such as thinning of its walls, dryness, and irritation.
- **Postmenopausal weight gain:** During menopause, the decrease in estrogen levels may increase the likelihood of weight gain. However, it's important to know that low estrogen isn't the sole cause—aging, lifestyle choices, and genetics also contribute. As people get older, they tend to lose muscle and gain more fat.

REASSURANCE AMIDST MENOPAUSAL CHANGES

Despite the changes brought by menopause, you must understand that it is normal to experience these issues—and you're not alone.

Seeking support from healthcare professionals, friends, or support groups can provide valuable guidance and reassurance during this new phase of life.

The DUTCH Test

The DUTCH test is a hormonal panel used to assess hormonal imbalance in all stages of reproduction—from perimenopause to postmenopause. If you are a woman using hormone replacement therapy, this test is a helpful way to check the levels of the hormones you are taking. This test is especially good for monitoring oral progesterone, hormone creams applied vaginally, patches, and pellets.

The DUTCH test also keeps an eye on your melatonin levels. Melatonin is a hormone produced in your body about two hours before bedtime, and it helps you feel relaxed and sleepy. If you're having trouble sleeping, knowing your melatonin levels could be useful in figuring out the right treatment for you (*Top 5 Reasons You Should Be Using The DUTCH Test*, n.d.).

Female Hormone Test

A female hormone test looks at all your hormones and gives your doctor a clear idea of how they are doing and what their current levels are. These hormones include estrogen, progesterone, follicle-stimulating hormone, testosterone, and thyroid hormones.

It's best to take your hormonal test results to a healthcare provider. Although it's good to know about your hormones, only a doctor can provide a comprehensive health plan according to your reports.

KEY TAKEAWAYS

Menopause and the symptoms it comes with are completely normal for all women to go through. As a woman, embracing these changes can make it easier to deal with this new phase of your life.

Remember, you must understand where your symptoms are coming from and not fight them. As we move to the next chapter, we'll be talking about something that affects our health more than we may realize: food.

2

GOOD FOOD

Elsie, a woman in her early 50s, suddenly found herself disliking all the foods she used to love. She was quick to blame menopause for the drastic change and how nothing seemed appealing to her about food anymore. But worst of all, she found planning her daily meals a hassle, which led to her developing bad eating habits. She wanted to remain healthy, but she also felt like she lacked the energy and desire to focus on better eating habits. So, she often turned to convenience foods and sugar-laden snacks at the last minute.

If you can relate to that story, I'm sure you must have thought to yourself once in a while, *Why should I eat good food when I don't feel like eating anything at all? Why should I look after my nutritional values after being hit by menopause?*

Don't worry, in this chapter, you'll be taught how hydration and a balanced diet are keys to overall well-being, especially during menopause. You will also learn how they can help you manage your menopausal symptoms efficiently. So, let's get into it without further ado!

THE ROLE OF NUTRITION IN MENOPAUSE

Nutrition plays a vital role while recovering or going through the fluctuating changes of menopause. Eating a balanced diet during menopause gives you all the nutrients you need. It helps you maintain a healthy weight. Apart from that, you can also reduce your risk of certain health problems that become inevitable, such as cardiovascular diseases and osteoporosis (*Learning About Healthy Eating During Menopause*, n.d.).

Taking in the right foods can help ease your menopause symptoms by supporting good digestion, maintaining the required amounts of important nutrients, and providing enough minerals, vitamins, and antioxidants to keep your body functioning at its best.

And can you guess the best part? Having a healthy diet as an integral part of your routine can also boost your self-confidence and outlook on life!

Dietary Choices in Menopause

Have you ever heard the common phrase, "You are what you eat"? When it comes to certain situations, such as menopause, this saying truly holds a lot of value. The following are some dietary choices (with their benefits) you should opt for during menopause. These are simple choices that will go a long way in supporting your menopause journey:

- **Dairy products:** Due to the lack of estrogen in your body, you become prone to fractures because of the decrease in bone density. Adequate intake of calcium, vitamins K and D, and dairy products such as yogurt, cheese, milk, phosphorus, potassium, and magnesium is necessary for maintaining strong and healthy bones. A 2017 study of women in postmenopause showed that the ones who consumed dairy and animal protein had better bone density than the ones who didn't (Palladino & Brown, 2018).

- **Whole grains, fruits, and vegetables:** Menopausal women are at a risk of having high cholesterol and heart disease. So, a heart-healthy diet that contains whole grains, fruits, vegetables, and lean proteins can help support cardiovascular health.
- **Phytoestrogen:** Phytoestrogen, found in foods such as soy products and flax seeds, acts as a weak estrogen in the body. It may help in managing hormonal imbalance and offer ease from menopausal symptoms.
- **Isoflavones:** Certain plant-based foods contain isoflavones, which act like a mild form of estrogen in the body. They are found in foods such as soybeans, chickpeas, pistachios, and peanuts. These foods might assist in reducing cholesterol levels and have been proposed to alleviate symptoms like hot flashes and night sweats (Johnson, 2022).
- **Foods to limit:** Avoid foods that are highly processed and have added sugars. such as soda. Limit alcohol, high-salt foods, and caffeine, as they are known to cause hot flashes and night sweats.

Important Nutrients During Menopause

Now that we have discussed necessary dietary choices, let's talk about important nutrients that are helpful for your body during menopause in detail:

- **Calcium and vitamin D:** Calcium is important to maintain bone density, as a lack of estrogen can make the bones brittle and weak. A good source of calcium and vitamin D can be yogurt. Intake of calcium also prevents osteoporosis. Other sources include leafy green vegetables, tofu, almonds, and fatty fish such as salmon and mackerel (Upham & Franco, 2023).

- **Protein:** Protein is essential for muscle maintenance and repair. It also plays a vital part in weight management, as it provides the feeling of fullness and supports lean muscle mass. Good sources of protein are lean meats, poultry, fish, nuts, seeds, and eggs.

- **Omega-3s:** Omega-3 fatty acids, specifically EPA (eicosapentaenoic acid) and DHA (docosahexaenoic acid) have anti-inflammatory properties. They can help reduce inflammation, alleviate joint pain, and may also contribute to mood stability. Good sources of omega-3s are chia seeds, walnuts, and fish oil supplements.

- **Magnesium:** Magnesium is involved in various biochemical processes in the body, such as bone health, muscle function, and nerve function. It can also help alleviate symptoms such as muscle cramps. Good sources of magnesium are green veggies, nuts, whole grains, and legumes.

Changes in Metabolism and Weight Management

If you've experienced menopause or menopause symptoms, I'm sure you must have thought, *Why can't I get rid of this tough belly fat?*

During menopause, many women complain of unwanted weight gain around the abdomen area. Apart from hormonal changes and declining estrogen levels, other factors can contribute to weight gain, including age, lifestyle changes, and genetic factors (*The Reality of Menopause Weight Gain*, 2023).

Some menopausal symptoms such as a poor sleep schedule, hot flashes, and bad mood swings can make it harder than usual to exercise regularly and eat healthy food, which can eventually lead to weight gain.

The fat around your abdomen is known as "visceral fat." This fat is unhealthy, as it can cause increased heart disease, type 2 diabetes, breast cancer, and even dementia. It may also worsen the hot flashes you are going through (*Menopause and Weight*, n.d.).

CREATING A MENOPAUSE-FRIENDLY DIET

Before I tell you how to create a menopause-friendly diet, it's more important that you take a hormone level test to determine how you can deal with a hormonal imbalance. Talk to a healthcare provider first, and you'll get a better idea of what areas you'd have to work on.

- **Reduce caffeine, alcohol, and spicy foods:** No matter how much you love these food items or can't seem to start your day without them, to deal with those hot flashes, you'll have to cut out caffeine and spicy hot sauces from your diet. In addition, unchecked levels of alcohol intake can cause not only hot flashes but also liver damage, heart disease, and certain types of cancer. Make sure to consume these items in moderation.
- **Meet all magnesium needs:** Menopause can cause insomnia in some women. Although there is no scientific research to support magnesium supplement intakes, you should try to meet your magnesium needs by including it in your diet. For example, focus on getting enough whole grains, pumpkin seeds, almonds, and beans.

- **Include more phytoestrogens:** Phytoestrogens are substances found in plants that are kind of like human estrogen but not as strong. They have a similar structure and some similar effects but are generally less potent. They are also known to target hot flashes. Food sources of phytoestrogens are tofu, flax seeds, berries, apples, rice, and carrots.
- **Include lean proteins in every meal:** When it comes to proteins, choose lean meats and proteins to improve your menopause symptoms. This change can assist with managing weight, and it also makes sure your bones become more solid and your muscles become stronger.
- **Focus on calcium-rich foods:** You might not notice it immediately, but there's an increased risk of losing bone density during this period, which can eventually lead to conditions such as osteoporosis. To combat this, you must eat calcium-rich foods.
- **Get more vitamin D:** Vitamin D is necessary to absorb that calcium intake. So, you should always remember to pair your calcium-rich foods with vitamin D supplements to ensure better health.
- **Make sure that half your plate is veggies and fruits:** Vegetables and fruits are packed with the nutrition your body craves, as they promote good health. Choose colorful vegetables and fruits to make your meals more enjoyable, diverse, and nutritious.
- **Avoid extra fat:** Don't flush your healthy eating habits down the drain by including extra fat. For example, if you are having broccoli, don't pair it with a heavy gravy or melted cheese. Instead, you can add a punch of lemon zest and enjoy a lighter option.
- **Don't forget the dairy:** Dairy aids in maintaining your bone health, so don't sideline it from your meals

completely. Ensure you drink a glass of low-fat milk—or soy milk if you don't want to drink regular cow's milk. Just make sure to have a dairy source in the mix.

Importance of Hydration

What if I told you that incorporating one change in your entire routine would do wonders for your menopausal symptoms? I know I would do it, and that is why I want you to do it, too. Plus, it's pretty accessible and found in every household. Yes. I am talking about water.

Around 60% of our bodies are water (*The Water in You*, n.d.). Drinking healthy amounts of water will improve your skin, aid in better nails, improve brain function, reduce chances of urinary problems, relieve hot flashes, reduce headaches, and ease menopause cramps.

If you are exercising but not keeping yourself hydrated, chances are you will get dehydrated pretty quickly. To keep your body functioning at its peak, you must ensure that you are drinking at least eight glasses of water every day.

Staying hydrated in menopause is equally important. Water contains minerals that our brains and bodies need. If you don't love the taste of plain water, it's also good to know that fresh fruits and vegetables can also provide some of the hydration your body requires.

Meal Planning Tips

If you are a working woman, a busy stay-at-home mom, or someone who finds meal planning stressful, here are some helpful tips for you to follow:

- **Plan once for the whole week:** Set aside some time when you can plan your meals for the week. It doesn't matter if it is a weekday or weekend, just ensure that it's a consistent time that works for you.
- **Eat the same foods on different days of the week:** Decide a theme for what you are going to eat every day. For example: Meat Monday or Fish Friday. This can help you stay creative.
- **Monitor what you have at home:** Keep track of what ingredients are available in your pantry. This will help you save money, not overspend, and stop wasting food.
- **Find simple recipes:** Look for recipes online and choose the ones that take less time and are easy to prepare. Visit the supermarket with a list that has the exact proportions of things you need to buy.
- **Try new things and prep beforehand:** Don't be afraid to try something new—just save them for the weekend or when you have time. Prep the vegetables or marinate the chicken beforehand so you don't have to do it last minute.

The Gut Zoomer Test

In the United States, around 60 to 70 million people are affected by digestive diseases that result in millions of visits to the doctor (Cloyd, 2023). The Gut Zoomer Test is a comprehensive gut health test offered by the company called Vibrant Wellness. It is designed to assess the health of your gut microbiome, which refers to the trillions of microorganisms living in your digestive tract. The report comes with easy-to-read reports that can empower health-care providers to formulate personalized dietary, supplement, and lifestyle recommendations for their patients.

If you have digestive issues or unexplained symptoms such as skin problems or lack of energy—or even if you just want to support your overall well-being—you should consider taking this test and discussing the results with your healthcare provider.

How to Read Food Labels

Reading food labels is important when it comes to making healthy and informed choices. Ensure you stick to the following pointers to make a better decision.

- **Pay attention to the ingredients list:** Choose products that have recognizable foods with shorter ingredient lists. Ingredients are usually listed in descending order according to weight. Ensure you pay attention to the first few ingredients, as they usually make up most of the whole product.
- **Check out the serving size:** Look out for the serving size mentioned on the label. All the information regarding the nutrients is based on the serving size.
- **Note the nutrition facts:** Pay attention to the nutrients, such as calories, saturated fat, total fat, trans fat, sodium, cholesterol, fibers, total carbohydrates, and proteins. When you are aiming for a healthy diet, opt for foods that limit or don't have sodium, saturated and trans fat, and cholesterol.
- **Watch out for added sugars:** Choose products that have low sugar. Don't buy the ones that have added sugars or total sugars. Don't be fooled by other names for sugar, such as high fructose, sucrose, corn syrups, etc.
- **Be mindful of allergens:** Look out for products that have certain ingredients that could flare your allergies. Even if

you are only sensitive to certain ingredients, it's best to avoid those food items.

- **Check for expiration dates:** Ensure that the product you are buying is within the expiration date to ensure freshness and safety. Choose options that go well with your health goals. It's also best to compare similar products before making a final choice.

Tips on Eating Out

Eating out once in a while is something all of us enjoy. Just because you are taking care of your diet while going through menopause doesn't mean you don't get to enjoy dining out!

However, there are some tips you should be mindful of. Adhere to the following and you'll not only enjoy your night out but will also stick to your health goals:

- **Ask for more vegetables:** It's easier to get swayed when you're out to eat and those aromas are making your stomach rumble. However, do your best to stick to your nutritional goals. Instead of ordering something unhealthy, ask for more vegetables instead.
- **Go for whole grains:** Including a variety of whole grains in your diet provides essential nutrients such as fiber, vitamins, minerals, and antioxidants. Instead of ordering regular rice, go for brown rice instead. It's an easy swap!
- **Keep sodium (salt) in check:** Restaurant foods often have an alarming amount of salt. Be mindful of the food you are ordering and ask for options with minimal salt.
- **Get sauce and dressings on the side:** Sauces and dressing can add a lot more fat to your meal than there already is. To avoid that from happening, ask for them on the side of

your plate so you can better control how much you are eating.

- **Skip drinks with added sugar:** Drinking beverages that have a lot of added sugar can increase your risk of type 2 diabetes and obesity (West, 2017). So, to keep yourself on the safe side, go for unsweetened drinks or water.

INTERMITTENT FASTING AND KETO

Intermittent fasting and keto are two of the current health trends that have been tried and tested by many people. You have probably heard about them. Let's discuss what they are all about and how you can start incorporating them to support your body during menopause.

Intermittent Fasting

Intermittent fasting is basically limiting yourself to eat during designated hours. There are several variations of intermittent fasting that you can opt for depending on your choice.

- **The daily method:** The most popular method of intermittent fasting is the daily method. It follows the 16/8 or 18/6 rule. This means eating your regular food within a 6–8 hour timeframe each day and then fasting the remaining hours. The daily method is said to be the best method for intermittent fasting. For beginners, you can even eat during a 12-hour timeframe and then fast for the remaining 12 hours. Remember to start hydrating with water early. Drinking 8 ounces of water on an empty stomach will detoxify your body first thing in the morning.

- **The 24-hour method:** This method is a stricter one. It involves fasting for an entire day before you start eating again. Although it is done once or twice a week and people skip from breakfast to breakfast or lunch to lunch, this method is not recommended. This is because it can come along with fatigue, extreme headaches, and moodiness. Try to stick to the daily method before going for the 24-hour method.
- **Alternate method:** Choosing this method can do wonders, as you can eat normally every other day. On the days you are fasting, you can eat only 25% of what you were eating daily.

As for women going through menopause, intermittent fasting poses loads of benefits—and not just for weight loss. Fasting has been shown to promote hormone secretion from the thyroid. This can prevent bone problems such as osteoporosis and lower back pain (Brennan, 2021). Moreover, it can also reduce brain fog and improve mental clarity, increase energy, detoxify your system, and balance your sex hormones.

Intermittent fasting can also help boost your metabolism and decrease your blood pressure and even that rigid belly fat that comes along as women hit menopause. It also helps with your mental and physical health.

However, before you start following any of these methods, you need to know that intermittent fasting is not for everyone. If you have a history of eating disorders or are suffering from a medical condition, it's better to consult a doctor first. You should always prioritize your overall health instead of focusing only on weight loss.

Keto Diet

The ketogenic, or keto, diet is a high-fat, low-carbohydrate diet that often results in weight loss. The goal is to put the body in a state of ketosis, meaning that the body uses fat for energy, turning it into ketones (Jones, 2022).

Although a keto diet is known to help you reduce weight, the effects on menopause have been a little less clear. However, it is said to decrease your weight gain, control your cravings, and balance insulin levels.

If you are wondering whether keto can bring you out of menopause, the answer is no. No supplement, no diet, nothing can bring you out of menopause. Menopause is a natural process that occurs in every woman, and it cannot be stopped.

To start a keto diet, you can follow the tips listed below:

- **Consult a doctor:** Before you make any significant changes to your diet, especially if you have any preexisting conditions, it is best to consult a doctor. They can aid you in creating a personalized plan.
- **Plan your meals:** Plan your meals so you can ensure that you're getting the right amount of macronutrients. Include healthy fats, protein, and low-carb vegetables.
- **Shop for keto-friendly items:** Make a list of keto-friendly items that you would like to add to your diet and stock up on them. This may include meat, eggs, dairy products, etc.
- **Get rid of high-carb foods:** Clear out any high-carb foods from your pantry and refrigerator to avoid any sort of temptation. Cravings can get the best of us all, and it is better to be safe than sorry. Discard or donate the items that are not aligned with your keto diet.

- **Be mindful of "keto flu":** Some people following the keto diet may experience headaches and fatigue in the first few days. This phase is often referred to as the "keto flu." To avoid such problems, keep yourself hydrated and ensure you consume a sufficient amount of electrolytes to alleviate any symptoms.

Good vs. Bad Fats in Keto

While sticking to a keto diet, you must understand that not every kind of fat is healthy. Below are some kinds of fats you should avoid as much as you can while sticking to a keto diet:

Bad Fats

- **Artificial trans fats:** Artificial trans fat is a type of unsaturated fat that is chemically altered through a process called hydrogenation. During this process, hydrogen is added to the liquid vegetable oils to make them solid at room temperature and improve the texture of the food. Steering clear of foods labeled as trans-fat-free can be challenging, as products listing hydrogenated or partially hydrogenated oils may still contain trans fats. Despite the difficulty in complete avoidance, it is essential to invest time in scrutinizing nutrition facts and ingredients to reduce trans fat intake.
- **Highly processed fats:** When fats go through a lot of processing and get heated at very high temperatures, they can be bad for your health. Heating these fats creates harmful substances called free radicals, which can damage your body and cause inflammation. Processed oils often have a lot of omega-6 fatty acids, and having too many of these can be risky. Research suggests that consuming too many omega-6 fatty acids increases the chances of getting

heart disease and other long-term health problems (Nalwoga, n.d.).

- **Deep-fried foods:** When you deep-fry, you cook food in oil that's heated to 350 °F (175 °C) or even higher. At these high temperatures, the oil changes, creating harmful free radicals. In restaurants, the same oil is often used many times before they replace it.

Good Fats

Now, let's get to know about the good fats you should stick with while following a keto diet:

- **Saturated fats:** Saturated fats are healthy for your body. Since they are different from other fats, they don't have certain types of molecular bonds called double bonds. The lack of double bonds makes saturated fats more stable and less likely to go through a process called oxidation.
- **Monounsaturated fats:** Monounsaturated fats are fats that have only one double carbon bond in their molecular structure. It is said that they decrease the risk of cardiovascular diseases. Monounsaturated fats may help improve cholesterol levels and provide other health benefits when consumed in moderation.
- **Polyunsaturated fats:** Polyunsaturated fats are a type of dietary fat that contains multiple double bonds in their molecular structure. These fats are considered essential because our bodies cannot produce them naturally, so we need to obtain them from our diet. Two main types of polyunsaturated fats are omega-3 fatty acids and omega-6 fatty acids.

Keto-Friendly Recipes to Try

You can try any of these seven keto-friendly suggestions. When you are following a keto diet, you can enjoy them without the fear of gaining unwanted weight:

- **Keto snack bars:** These are the perfect snacks you can opt for if you are craving something sweet. They don't have any gluten or dairy.
- **Keto fish and chips:** Use almond meal instead of breadcrumbs and avocado instead of potatoes. You don't have to miss out on fish and chips now.
- **Keto taco shells:** You can make these easy spinach taco shells in the comfort of your home if you want to have Mexican food for dinner.
- **Keto chow mein:** You can add zucchini noodles to this classical Asian twist and there you have it. Your keto-friendly chow mein is ready to eat.
- **Keto eggs with salmon:** Out of breakfast ideas? You can make delicious eggs in a pot with salmon. Enjoy this gooey dish with a piece of keto-friendly bread, too.
- **Cream of cauliflower soup:** This is the perfect recipe to try in winter. It's easy, yummy, and vegetarian—just the right food for a keto diet.
- **Spiced almonds:** Looking for a spicy snack? Go for spiced almonds. They not only provide the nutrition but also that kick of spice you're looking for.

If you are looking to combine both keto and intermittent fasting, you can go for it since it is a safe option. However, if you have a history of eating disorders or a medical condition that may prevent you from following these diets, then it's best to refer to your doctor for specialized recommendations.

Monitoring Macros

Tracking macros (macronutrients) on the keto diet involves monitoring your daily intake of carbohydrates, fats, and proteins. Follow these steps to ensure you are monitoring your macros the right way:

- **Set the macronutrient goals:** Determine your daily goals based on your activity, individual needs, and health goals. In a standard keto diet, the macronutrient breakdown is often around 70% to 80% of calories from fat, 20% to 25% from protein, and 5% to 10% from carbohydrates.
- **Use an app or tool:** You can use a tracking app or tool to keep better track of your macros. You can choose from a variety of macro-tracking apps, including Lumen, MyFitnessPal, Lifesum, FatSecret, or MyMacros+.
- **Read nutrition labels:** Be aware of the nutrition labels on packaged foods to determine their macronutrient count. Pay attention to the hidden carbs and added sugars, as they can impact your daily carbohydrate intake and have the potential to keep you from reaching your goals.
- **Adjust portions:** If your macros are not aligning with the goals you have set, it's time to review and adjust your portions. This may involve increasing or decreasing the desired nutrients in your food.
- **Stay consistent:** Consistency is key when it comes to anything in your life. Make sure that you give the process time and stay consistent with the goals you have set. Make it a habit to log in your meals and remember that change takes place over time, not overnight.

Alternatives to the Keto Diet

If you don't want to follow a keto diet, here are some other options you can consider:

- **Zero-carb diet:** A zero-carb diet means that you only eat meat and fat. This type of diet can aid in weight loss, control your blood sugar, and balance your appetite control. However, it is also considered an extremely risky choice, as this option lacks some key nutrients, may cause digestive issues, and can even cause keto flu.
- **The South Beach diet:** The South Beach diet is a popular commercial diet plan designed to promote weight loss. It is a widely followed diet because it is divided into three phases, which makes the transition phase easier. It focuses on healthy fats and carbs while promoting blood sugar regulation. However, many people may find purchasing specific South Beach diet-branded products can be costly compared to regular grocery shopping.
- **Low-carb Mediterranean diet:** A low-carb Mediterranean diet reduces the intake of carbohydrates and is rich in fruits, vegetables, and healthy fats. It is said to promote heart health, is sustainable, and helps in shedding those pounds. Nevertheless, it has some potential nutrient gaps, can influence keto flu, and is complex due to the restrictions in meal planning. It can also prove to be socially difficult, as dining out can be an issue, and not a lot of restaurants offer Mediterranean diet options (Migala & Anderson, 2023).

SUPPLEMENTS AND MENOPAUSE

A balanced diet consists of consuming the right amounts of vegetables, carbs, protein, and fats to help keep your menopause symptoms in check. However, at times you may need an extra boost from various supplements to keep yourself healthy and strong.

The goal is to ensure that your body receives the correct amount of nutrition. When you enter perimenopause or menopause, you may need a boost as your estrogen levels drop and your metabolism slows down (*Best Supplements for Menopause*, 2022).

Supplements That are Beneficial for Menopause

Let's talk about the common supplements and herbs that can make menopause a smoother journey:

- **Calcium and vitamin D:** Bone health can become a serious concern once menopause strikes and your hormone level drops. Women require around 1,200 grams of calcium in their bodies each day, and this level must be maintained (Satmary & Dresden, 2021). Calcium and vitamin D promote bone health and density. If you require supplements to meet your intake needs, ensure that you take them in small doses with your food during the day.
- **Red clover:** Although red clover is a popular option for women to take when their estrogen levels drop, it is not proven scientifically. The research opinions have remained mixed over the years. Talk to your doctor before making any decision about using this supplement.
- **Ginseng:** A study proved that ginseng might help improve quality of life, especially for women who are going

through menopause. The study claimed that ginseng has a soothing effect on sexual function and hot flashes (Johnson, 2022).

- **Black cohosh:** Black cohosh is a common herb for menopausal symptoms. Native Americans traditionally used this plant to help with issues such as fever, cough, and irregular menstruation. European settlers also used this plant to support women's reproductive health. It is said to battle hot flashes, vaginal dryness, and irritability.

Although calcium and vitamin D are keto-friendly supplements, you can also opt for magnesium and omega-3 fatty acids (Kubala, 2018).

However, before you start any supplement or herbal regimen, you must choose the ones that are of the highest quality. If you don't know what to incorporate into your diet or don't know how to find the supplements that will benefit you, consult your healthcare provider or your doctor to ensure your safety.

Maintaining a healthy diet and taking care of your nutritional values during menopause is vital to ensure a better quality of life. Now that we have explored the benefits and sources of good food to include in your diet, let's talk about another important factor of your well-being: sleep!

3

RESTORATIVE SLEEP

Apart from the good, nutritious food you need during menopause, getting quality sleep is critical, too. There is simply no way to effectively manage your menopause symptoms and overall health without getting a good night's sleep. In this chapter, we will navigate how menopause affects sleep, what to do about it, and how you can incorporate healthier options into your schedule.

Although we already know that a lack of consistent patterns of quality sleep during menopause can cause hot flashes, did you know that it can also contribute to depression and might cause you to become more forgetful (*Sleep Problems and Menopause*, 2021)? These are only a few of the problems that come with a lack of restful, restorative sleep.

UNDERSTANDING SLEEP CHALLENGES DURING MENOPAUSE

As we know, menopausal symptoms can vary from woman to woman; however, it is no surprise that menopause is a time of hormonal, physical, and physiological change for women, which can deeply impact sleep quality.

Apart from the frustrating weight gain, mood shifts, and low sex drive, something else most women don't even think about is also affected during menopause: sleep. Some women need less sleep than others and vice versa; however, a healthy sleep cycle consists of somewhere from seven to eight hours per night, although it's not a hard and fast rule (Pien, n.d.). You can experiment with what works for you—just remember to aim for at least this amount as a goal.

Did you also know that as women enter their late 40s and early 50s, the number of sleep complaints jumps from 12% to 40% (*How Can Menopause Affect Sleep?* 2022)?

Common Sleep Issues During Menopause

Now that we understand how menopause can affect your sleep cycle, let's talk about the common sleep issues that may inevitably occur.

- **Hot flashes:** The majority of the time, women feel sleepless because of hot flashes. These unpleasant feelings may pop up from time to time and at any given time during the day or night. They are hot and unexpected sensations that happen all over your body and can cause sweating, too. At night, a hot flash can wake you up and ruin your sleep in the process. Before a hot flash strikes, your body temperature rises, and heat travels all the way to your face, creating a sensation that wakes you up—even the act of getting up to use the bathroom can initiate a hot flash.

- **Insomnia:** Insomnia is described as a condition where individuals find chronic difficulty falling or staying asleep. This occurs three or more times a week. People with insomnia don't sleep well; they might toss and turn, wake up too early, and feel tired during the day. Not getting enough sleep can make them feel more anxious and irritable, affect their ability to concentrate and remember things, and lead to more headaches and inflammation. Women who are going through menopause may experience insomnia due to hot flashes and night sweats.

- **Other sleep disorders:** Along with hot flashes and insomnia, other sleep disorders such as sleep apnea and snoring are common, too. Sleep apnea is a potentially serious disorder in which the breathing repeatedly stops and starts. The main types of sleep apnea are obstructive sleep apnea (OSA) and central sleep apnea (CSA). If you snore too loudly or happen to feel tired even after a full night's sleep, you may have sleep apnea (*Sleep Apnea - Symptoms and Causes*, 2023). If you have concerns, it is best to consult with your healthcare provider.

Role of Estrogen and Progesterone

Fluctuating levels of estrogen and progesterone during menopause can affect your sleep cycle, too.

Estrogen, which is the main female sex hormone, is responsible for controlling a woman's menstruation cycle, whereas progesterone helps in maintaining pregnancy; meaning that its levels are the highest during that time. These hormones fluctuate at various stages of a woman's life, including during menopause, and because of that, sleep quality is affected, too. Women often complain of hot flashes during menopause and report poor sleep, and fluctuating hormones could be the culprit (*Which Hormones Affect Sleep?* 2022).

Remember that if you have any concerns regarding your sleep, or if you find yourself often disturbed and uncomfortable because of your symptoms, you should visit a doctor immediately. Don't wait for the intensity of your symptoms to heighten to the point that they start interfering with your daily life. If you feel exhausted and fatigued or feel like skipping out on your responsibilities, see a doctor as soon as you can.

SETTING THE STAGE FOR BETTER SLEEP

For you to get those optimal hours of sleep, it's imperative to begin with the right settings for your bedroom. Follow these tips to create an environment that is more conducive to sleep and to help yourself get better sleep during menopause:

- **Darken your room:** Light is known to slow down the production of melatonin, a naturally occurring hormone that is responsible for promoting sleep. Make sure to make your bedroom darker either by lowering your shades or having black-out curtains. Start dimming the lights in your bedroom as nighttime approaches. Wrap up any work you have to create a good environment to sleep in. Turn off your cell phone and TV to limit your exposure to blue light. You can also set your devices to night mode since continued exposure to light can keep you awake and disrupt your sleep. It's better to stay away from your devices at least one hour before you go to sleep.
- **Lower the temperature:** Experts agree that the perfect temperature to fall asleep is somewhere between 60 °F to 67 °F for quality sleep (*How to Make a Sleep-Friendly*

Bedroom, 2020). As you fall asleep, your body temperature decreases to promote the sleep-inducing process. So, keeping your bedroom cool facilitates this natural occurrence and helps you fall asleep much easier. However, this temperature can be a bit chilly for some. But remember: If your hot flashes have made it impossible for you to sleep, maintaining this temperature might just do the trick.

- **Choose a comfortable mattress and sheet set:** Knowing what type of mattress, bed sheets, and pillows you require for a good night's sleep is vital if you want to rest peacefully. Your mattress choice is essential depending on the type of sleep position you prefer, whether you share a bed, or if you happen to "run hot" during the night. As for your pillows, if you choose the wrong ones, you may have neck problems and headaches. You must also consider what to put on top of your mattress. Opt for sheets that are pure cotton or any material that provides you with nothing less than the comfort you're looking for.

- **Reduce noise:** How can you expect a good night's sleep if it's not pin-drop silence in your bedroom? When it's time for bed, minimize all the unwanted noise that can potentially ruin your sleep. If you live in a busy neighborhood or near a busy street, consider getting your walls soundproofed. You can also adjust your bed away from the walls or windows to stop the noises to a certain level.

By following these tips, you'll be able to create the perfect environment for you to sleep soundly throughout the night. These changes can also help with your menopause symptoms such as night sweats, hot flashes, and insomnia.

Create Your Own Pre-Sleep Routine

If your menopause symptoms are causing a ruckus, it's best to come up with a pre-sleep routine. Use these tips to create a routine that works for you and then follow it every day, whether it is a weeknight or a weekend:

- **Food:** Avoid spicy food, as it can cause night sweats or hot flashes while you sleep. Likewise, you should also resist the temptation to consume caffeine and nicotine. These chemicals only make it harder for you to sleep.
- **Exercise:** Research has shown that women who were in menopause and performed regular aerobic exercises found it easier to sleep at night. They also found that their mood swings were balanced and they felt happier (Eiser, 2021). Try incorporating exercises into your daily routine. You can even perform your favorite routines at least three hours before you go to bed. However, don't exercise right before you go to bed.
- **Bedroom environment:** Ensure that you have a cooler temperature set in your bedroom, as it will help you fall asleep faster. It will also keep those hot flashes and night sweats at bay. Try cotton bed sheets for your mattress for a change. These are cooler and are good at wicking moisture.
- **Bedtime schedule:** If you have night sweats, take a cold shower. If not, take a warm shower instead. Don't eat, read, or use your devices in bed. Make sure you put all of that away once you're going to bed. Visit the restroom before you go to bed as well so you can stay in a continuous sleep cycle. Try to relax as you hit those pillows. Worrying about not sleeping is going to make it

worse for you to sleep. Take deep breaths to prevent further stress.

TECHNIQUES FOR RELAXATION AND IMPROVED SLEEP

Stress and anxiety can often make it harder for us to fall and remain asleep. Many people struggle to fall asleep, and it's quite common for women during menopause, as we know. Even if we don't have insomnia, many of us can relate to the difficulty of getting some shut-eye, especially after a stressful day.

You must include healthy sleeping habits to ensure you can sleep peacefully without being disrupted. If you create your own pre-sleep routine and still find it difficult to fall asleep, you can apply these techniques for additional relaxation and improved sleep hygiene.

Breathing Exercises

Taking long, slow breaths is the most simple way to feel relaxed and connected with your body. If you are struggling to fall asleep and find yourself lying awake in your bed, start by taking 10 deep breaths. This alone will help to calm you down. If you want to try any more breathing exercises, you can try the following suggestions to find what works best for you:

Diaphragmatic breathing: Also known as belly breathing or abdominal breathing, diaphragmatic breathing is a process where you engage the diaphragm muscle to promote relaxation and enhance oxygen intake, all of which is helpful for a restful night's sleep. Follow these steps:

1. Start by either sitting or lying down in a comfortable position. As we're trying to help you sleep, do this while you are in your bedroom.
2. Put one hand on your chest and the other on your abdomen. This will help you be aware of your breathing and where it is originating from.
3. Breathe in slowly through your nose, allowing the air to fill in your lungs. Focus on feeling your abdomen rise and ensure that your chest stays firm.
4. Exhale slowly through your mouth. Pay attention to the sensation of your abdomen. Your exhale should take longer than your inhale.
5. Incorporate diaphragmatic breathing into your daily routine. Aim to do it a few times throughout the day but especially before going to bed.

4-7-8 breathing: This type of breathing exercise is also known as the relaxing breath, which is a simple yet effective method used to promote relaxation and reduce stress levels. This is how it's done:

1. Get in a comfortable position. Ensure your back is straight and your shoulders are relaxed.
2. Place the tip of your tongue on the roof of your mouth. Keep it just behind your upper front teeth. Keep your tongue in a position like this throughout the whole exercise.
3. Exhale completely to ensure that there is no air left in your lungs.
4. Close your mouth and inhale quietly through your nose, counting to four in your mind. Focus on taking a slow and deep breath, allowing your abdomen to expand.

5. After inhaling, hold your breath for a count of seven. This step helps to oxygenate your blood and allows the breath to be absorbed fully.

6. Open your mouth slightly and exhale completely while counting to eight.

Repeat this exercise whenever you feel stressed or can't seem to fall asleep. This technique is a helpful tool to ensure that you stay calm even if you're feeling stressed.

Visualization Exercises

You can also use visualization exercises, which are great for your overall well-being, and use mental images to reduce stress and help you fall asleep. This is a type of meditation that is a good alternative or complement to breathing exercises.

Body scan: Body scans are a type of meditation that is done to bring present-time awareness to your body.

1. Start to relax yourself by diaphragmatic or 4-7-8 breathing to slow down.

2. Bring your attention to a specific body part, noticing any sensations and seeing if you are holding any tension in this part of your body.

3. If you notice any discomfort, acknowledge it and let go of any stories or incidents related to it. Visualize the tension leaving your body.

4. You can visualize the tension and sensations leaving your body through breathing.

5. Move your attention to each part of your body until you are done scanning your whole body, starting from the feet

and moving to the forehead. Continue doing it until you feel like all the tension has been released.

Autogenic training: Autogenic training takes you through the same steps as a body scan. The only additions are the statements you make about the heaviness and sensations in your body. With practice, you will be able to calm down any part of your body (*Relaxation Exercises to Help Fall Asleep*, 2023).

If you find it too distracting or difficult to remember what statements you said how many times, you can either record yourself or find supportive audio recordings on the internet as well.

Progressive Muscle Relaxation

Progressive muscle relaxation (PMR) is a successful tool also used to manage stress, help you sleep better, and promote deeper, uninterrupted sleep.

The goal of progressive muscle relaxation is to squeeze and clench each of your muscles as you breathe in and release tension as you breathe out. It works best when you're lying in bed at night and also first thing in the morning (Bygraves & Witton, 2021). Follow these steps to do it:

1. Clench each muscle in your body. Begin with your forehead and face, down your shoulders, your back, thighs, lower legs, and feet.
2. Remember to breathe in as you clench and breathe out as you let go.
3. Perform a scan of your body before and after to see what the results are and what differences you can feel.

Self-hypnosis: Self-hypnosis is similar to progressive muscle relaxation we just talked about. In this, you have to focus on specific thoughts with full concentration after you have relaxed.

The idea is that when your body is truly relaxed, it is open to more suggestions. Before you begin, think about what you want to focus on. You can either pick a word or a phrase that you can repeat while shifting your body toward muscle relaxation.

Once you get the hang of self-hypnosis, you can add other things little by little. You can picture yourself in a safer place. Try to imagine the sights, smells, and feelings surrounding you. For example, you can start by thinking you are in a beautiful space surrounded by things you love.

IMPORTANCE OF REGULAR SLEEP SCHEDULES

As we talked about, it is imperative to have healthy sleeping habits. In addition, it is also important to have regular sleep schedules to ensure your mental and physical state remains good.

You must ensure that you wake up and go to sleep at the same time. This reinforces your body's circadian rhythm, which can make it easier for you to sleep and wake up every day. Getting seven to eight hours of sleep is essential. So, whatever sleeping time you choose, make sure it falls within that range.

Try using your bed only for sleeping. Don't lie down on your bed if you aren't tired and just toss and turn. When you create a certain relationship with the things around you, then your body reacts the same way as well.

If you lie in your bed and can't seem to sleep after 20 minutes, wake up and do something until you fall asleep. You could read a book, do some chores, or even write down your feelings in a journal, as journaling can help you unwind your day.

If you still have insomnia even after creating healthy sleep habits and maintaining a regular sleep schedule, you can contact a healthcare provider to get better insights as to why you can't sleep. At times, it's better to get yourself checked before jumping to any conclusion.

Get in Touch With Your Circadian Rhythm

A circadian rhythm is a natural, internal process that regulates the sleep and wake cycle and repeats every 24 hours. It is often referred to as the body's biological clock. However, this rhythm is influenced by external factors such as light and darkness (*Can You Change Your Circadian Rhythm?* 2024).

Keep these key points in mind if you are thinking of altering your circadian rhythm:

- **Sleep-wake cycle:** The circadian rhythm plays an important role in determining when we feel asleep or awake throughout the day. It influences the timing of various bodily functions, such as body temperature, hormone production, and metabolism.
- **Light influence:** Exposure to natural light is crucial, as it is the primary factor that regulates circadian rhythms. Light signals are received by the eyes and communicate with the internal clock of the brain to synchronize your body's functions with the external environment. Red light can activate and deactivate melatonin in the brain. Rising early to see the sunrise and watching the sunset can set the stage for better sleep.

- **Melatonin:** Melatonin is a hormone that is responsible for making us sleepy. Melatonin levels rise in the evening as the darkness starts to prevail. It signals the body to start winding down so the body can go to sleep.
- **Impact on health:** Maintaining a cycle that aligns with a person's circadian rhythm is associated with better health. Chronic disruptions to circadian rhythms have been linked to sleep disorders, mood disorders, and various health issues.
- **Age-influenced changes:** Circadian rhythms can change with age. Adolescents often report a shift in their natural sleep-wake preferences, leading to a tendency to stay up later and sleep in.

Understanding our circadian rhythms can help us improve our sleep and overall well-being. However, it involves creating a consistent sleep schedule, getting exposure to sunlight, and having good sleep hygiene.

I hope the key strategies and insights we shared in this chapter gave you a profound insight into how to ensure that you sleep well, even when permanent shifts such as menopause show up.

Quality sleep is integral to overall health, and its importance becomes even more profound during menopause when sleep patterns are disrupted and symptoms such as hot flashes and night sweats show up in full swing.

In the next chapter, we will learn about staying active and how it can positively affect women during menopause.

4

STAYING ACTIVE

During menopause, along with proper food and adequate sleep, staying active is an imperative part of your journey, too. In this chapter, we'll explore the power of physical activities and how they enable us to remain in shape throughout menopause and aid our mental health as well.

A woman going through menopause found the courage and power to keep herself healthy and deal with the menopausal symptoms effectively. She found exercising as a way to release her endorphins and remain happy and energetic, even when the world gave her all the reasons to sulk away in stress and anxiety (*My Story: How Regular Exercise Helped Me Manage My Menopause Symptoms,* 2023). Let's look at how we can harness the same benefits:

THE POWER OF EXERCISE DURING MENOPAUSE

Undoubtedly, menopause is a major shift in a woman's life. Learning how to navigate the changes is key to managing your symptoms. Having to deal with your symptoms constantly on top of your roller coaster mood swings isn't the picture that most of us had in mind. However, we can still thrive and live life to the fullest by taking care of ourselves.

You might also wonder, *What is it that these women are doing that they aren't affected by menopause?* Well, the answer to that is simple: exercise.

Yes, you read that correctly. Exercise and menopause have a positive relationship. Exercise can help you alleviate your symptoms, and it can also improve the quality of your life overall.

Research showed differences between women who exercised during menopause and those who didn't. The ones who didn't exercise found their symptoms worse than the ones who did. The ones who did exercise saw a significant amount of change in their physical and mental health as well (Payne, 2021).

To better understand how physical activity helps you stay healthy during the demanding transition of menopause, let's look at some of the key advantages below:

- **Improves bone strength and health:** As menopause begins, your estrogen levels start to drop dramatically. Although bone density starts to decrease at the age of 30, your bone density reaches an increased risk of developing osteoporosis during your later years. Also known as brittle bones, osteoporosis can pose a concerning problem for menopausal women. However, once you start to exercise regularly, you can maintain and improve your bone density to an extent. You can improve your muscle strength and balance, which can also reduce your chances of tripping or falling.
- **Prevents weight gain:** Lack of estrogen can also cause you to lose muscle mass and gain abdominal mass. Not only

that, but lack of exercise and poor dietary choices contribute to weight gain as well. A complete exercise regimen and training can help you shed those unwanted pounds and maintain that lean muscle mass.

- **Reduces your risk of cancer:** You may be surprised to know that regular workouts throughout perimenopause and menopause are associated with reduced risks of certain types of cancer, including endometrial, colon, and breast cancers. It's important to note though that while working out can reduce the risk of cancers, it can't eliminate it. Your lifestyle factors have an influence as well, and risk factors such as family and genetics play a crucial role.

- **Reduces risk of other diseases:** Menopause can impact heart health and increase the risk of type 2 diabetes because of the extra weight gain that many women end up experiencing. Changes in cholesterol levels affect your heart and impair the body's ability to use insulin effectively. So, you can engage in regular exercise that will promote cardiovascular health and improve insulin sensitivity (*The Benefits of Exercise During Menopause*, 2015).

- **Combats stress:** If you've experienced them, it's no surprise to you that mood swings can be difficult to deal with. Menopausal symptoms become even harder to deal with because of fluctuating hormones. Exercising can help release endorphins, reduce cortisol levels, aid in muscle relaxation, and even improve your quality of sleep. In turn, all of this can help you manage your stress levels better.

- **Improves your mood:** Exercise has a profound impact on your mood and emotional well-being. Several mechanisms combine to produce positive effects of exercise on our mood. Engaging in regular physical activity can lead to various mental health benefits, such as reduced stress hormones, improved focus, boosted serotonin levels, increased energy levels, and enhanced self-esteem and confidence.

Exercises for Menopausal Needs

It's best to stick with a variety of exercises to ensure you hit all the goals you have in mind. You should aim for at least 30 minutes of exercise every day for five days a week (Wild, 2023).

Cardiovascular Exercises

Cardiovascular exercises, also known as cardio or aerobic exercises, are activities that increase your heart rate and breathing while keeping your large muscle groups engaged. These types of exercises are also known to improve your blood vessels and lung health.

Although everyone should perform regular workouts to stay healthy, women are at a greater risk of developing heart disease during menopause. The following exercises are great for your heart health:

- **Dancing:** Dancing is an excellent type of cardiovascular exercise that offers a combination of physical fitness. Not only that, but it also brings along a surge of enjoyment as well. It provides a full-body workout, engages various muscles, and boosts your heart health. Depending on the type and intensity of your dancing, you can burn a significant amount of calories, and this can contribute to your weight management. Regular dancing can improve your stamina and endurance over time. Your body becomes more efficient in taking oxygen, which is crucial for overall fitness.

- **Cycling:** If you compare high-impact exercises such as running with cycling, cycling is relatively gentler on the joints—which is something women need as they are going through menopause because it can affect bone density. In addition, cycling can have a positive impact on your mental well-being. It can reduce stress, anxiety, and depression while promoting a sense of freedom. Being outdoors in nature can help you connect with nature and provide vitamin D and a burst of fresh air.
- **High-intensity interval training:** High-intensity interval training (HIIT) is a form of cardiovascular exercise that shifts short, intense bursts of activity with periods of rest or lower-intensity exercise. The reason this training method has gained popularity is because of its short sessions as compared to a traditional cardio workout. It enhances metabolic function and has a variety of exercises to offer, which keeps boredom at bay and aids you in feeling better every time you come back to work out. It also helps increase aerobic capacity by lowering blood pressure.
- **Running:** One of the most popular and accessible forms of cardiovascular exercise that provides a wide range of physical and mental health benefits is running. Running allows you to reduce your risk of heart disease, and it also helps eliminate a condition known as brain fog (Cohen, 2022). It can improve your sleep cycle and boost your mood.

Strength Exercises

Due to the lack of estrogen after menopause, there is a risk of developing osteoporosis. This can lead to pain or an elevated risk of fractures. However, strength training can help you reduce that risk significantly. It can also keep you metabolically strong. To strength train, you can use free weights, gym machines, bands, or even your body weight.

You can use strength training to increase weight or resistance levels to strengthen your muscles and shed those extra pounds as well. Even if you feel anxious or are in a bad mood, strength training can help you out enormously.

- **Squats:** Squats make daily activities easier to perform because they mimic daily movements like standing and sitting. They are also beneficial for preventing age-related weight gain. Squats target the quadriceps, hamstrings, glutes, and calves, which can help in strengthening your lower body.
- **Planks:** Planks are perfect for strengthening the core muscles, including the abdominals and obliques. A strong core can improve your posture and reduce the risk of back pain as well. Holding a plank position also engages the muscles that contribute to balance and stability.
- **Push-ups:** Push-ups target the chest, shoulders, triceps, and upper back. Push-ups, like squats, put pressure on your bones, and this pressure can help keep your bones strong or make them even stronger. This is important during menopause when bone health becomes more significant. Remember that you can always do push-ups from your knees if you are a beginner or find it difficult.
- **Kettlebells, dumbbells, and other weights:** Lifting kettlebells, dumbbells, or other weights is a great way to strengthen your muscles and improve overall fitness. When you are incorporating weights into your routine, remember to start with ones you can easily carry and then

gradually increase the weight once your body becomes used to it.

- **Resistance-based gym machines:** During menopause, hormonal changes can cause a decrease in muscle mass. Doing exercises with resistance, like using gym machines, helps keep and even build muscle. This is important for staying strong and keeping a healthy metabolism, especially during menopause. Gym machines also provide stability, which is good for your joints. This can be helpful for women going through menopause who might feel some discomfort in their joints. If you are concerned about beginning a strength-training program, you can always consult your doctor first.

- **Yoga:** Taking a yoga class or simply rolling out your mat and doing a solo session can do wonders for you during menopause. It can help you lower your blood pressure and can also increase your flexibility and help you with your sleep.

- **Pilates:** If you don't want to do yoga, or if you want to try something refreshing, then you can also choose Pilates. Pilates places a strong emphasis on the core muscles, including the muscles of the abdomen, lower back, hips, and buttocks. Pilates exercises focus on doing movements with care and control. It's more about doing each movement correctly than doing a lot of them. People doing Pilates are encouraged to keep their bodies in the right position and do each exercise with good form. Pilates also emphasizes the connection between the mind and body. It is often used to promote mindfulness and concentration.

- **Tai chi:** Along with yoga and Pilates, tai chi also supports your balance and mobility. Tai chi is a traditional system of exercise that was developed in China in the 12th century. It was originally developed for the sake of self-defense and martial arts but slowly transitioned into a health and wellness practice (Migala & Laube, 2022). It involves a series of slow, graceful, and continuous movements. It emphasizes the connection between the mind and the body. Since it is considered a low-impact exercise, it is gentler on the body and can be done by women going through menopause, as they are at risk of brittle bones.

Walking

A lot of women going through menopause find it difficult to stick to a routine and go to the gym. One of the simplest ways to stay active and introduce exercise into your daily routine is by walking.

You might be wondering what benefits it poses for menopausal women, and you may be surprised to know that walking has a positive impact on your unpredictable menopause symptoms. Let's look at some of the ways walking can help you during menopause and how it can contribute to your overall health:

- **Boosts your immune system:** Did you know that walking daily for a moderate amount of time can help boost your immune system? It sounds too good to be true, but it is! As you walk every day, over time your immune and metabolic systems continue to strengthen, pump blood, and circulate your immune cells, which then help your body prepare better for a future infection. Alleviating your stress levels by walking also helps your immune system remain healthy (*Balance - 5 Reasons to Walk More During Menopause*, 2023).
- **Reduces risk of diseases and chronic conditions:** Research shows that walking can reduce your chances of getting breast cancer, especially during menopause, down to 20% to 30%. Another study proved that walking reduced

heart disease by 35%, according to an eight-year Harvard University study of more than 70,000 women ages 40 to 65 (Stanten & Linville, 2021).

- **Helps manage menopausal weight gain:** Walking can help you increase your metabolism rate, which in turn can help manage your menopausal weight gain. Doing something as simple as walking daily can affect your weight. A little bit of exercise accompanied by walking can help you burn calories. Moreover, we know how tough it is to deal with that dreaded belly fat, and walking can do wonders.

- **Improves your bone health:** When done at a brisk pace, walking is an excellent aerobic exercise that is good for your overall figure. Walking impacts your joints and lubricates them, which is good for your bone health. Sitting all day or not moving at all can stiffen your joints. So, the longer you walk, the more you let go of that stiffness and optimize muscle endurance and stamina (*7 Menopausal Benefits of a 10-Minute Walk*, 2019).

- **Supports your sleep cycle:** We know how hard it is to deal with those hot flashes and night sweats that make it feel impossible to sleep at night. However, walking can affect how well you sleep at night. When you perform any physical activity, your body needs time to rest up, so you feel the urge to sleep and recharge as well.

So, the next time you are thinking of skipping a day's walk, remind yourself how fruitful it will be for you in the long run.

BUILDING AND MAINTAINING EXERCISE MOTIVATION

I understand how hard it can be to exercise when menopause symptoms hit and you don't have the energy or feel like yourself. Digging deep for that motivation can be tough, but it's never impossible. Having the motivation and maintaining it over time can be achieved efficiently if you follow these tips:

- **Set SMART goals:** The SMART goal strategy is a popular method to maintain all your goals. It is known to work well for your fitness and has been broken down into the following key points:

  o Specific: Is your goal clear and defined?
  o Measurable: Can your goal be tracked?
  o Achievable: Is your goal doable?
  o Relevant: Is your goal relevant to your life purpose?
  o Timely: Can you decide on a date and hold accountable?

When followed, SMART goals can be super effective. They work best for those who are focused on the process rather than the outcome (*6 Expert Tips For Setting Realistic Fitness Goals,* 2023).

- **Use visualization to find your "why":** Visualizing the goals you have set for yourself can help you get started. This is a popular physiological technique that works well for your mind and body because it programs it to support your goal the way you want it. Whatever you are visualizing, ensure that it is something you are passionate about and are willing to process. If your goals don't align with your interests, visualizing them can be hard. Getting started with the SMART technique to help you find your "why."

- **Break down big goals into smaller parts:** If you set a big goal for yourself without breaking it down into smaller, accessible parts, you will likely grow tired of it and feel less motivated to continue. To keep yourself motivated, you must make those smaller parts of your goals, and once you achieve them, spoil yourself. Keep yourself focused on the big goal, but don't forget to appreciate the little stepping stones that come your way. They will make your goal more achievable and rewarding.

- **Create daily goal-supporting habits:** Write down your goal-supporting habits and follow them regularly. For example, if you achieved 300 steps today, add 50 more for tomorrow. Remaining focused throughout is a challenging task.

- **Create challenging but achievable goals:** If you are going to have goals that are too easy or are extremely unachievable, you won't be able to find a balance. Balance is important. Set goals for yourself that challenge and excite you to perform well. If you are ignoring your sleep and nutrition for your goal, that isn't healthy. Understand your abilities and set benchmarks for yourself. The more personal your goals are, the better you'll be able to complete them. Don't let someone else's progress influence you. Set a pace that is comfortable for you.

- **Enjoy the process:** If you do things you love, the process itself becomes enjoyable. If you continue thinking of your goals merely as things that you have to gain, you won't be able to smile and enjoy what you are doing. Remember, it doesn't matter if you are doing the smallest of your goals, what matters is that you enjoy the process.

- **Stay positive:** Nothing is going to happen overnight. You will not see any results in just a day or two. Give it time, stay positive, and remind yourself that you are doing a good job. Hype yourself up! Nothing is going to satisfy you more than being positive about what you are doing for yourself. Remind yourself to move forward, even if you feel like giving up.

You can begin by saying and committing to the following affirmations:

- I will exercise for 30 minutes three times a week.
- I will drink 6–8 glasses of water throughout the day.
- I will aim for 1,000 steps an hour.

Stick to these and you will find yourself motivated and willing to perform your fitness goals you've planned for yourself.

Engage Yourself

Start with physical activities you enjoy. If you love to walk your dog to the park, do it as a means to walk. If you like cycling to work, do it. If you like going hiking every weekend, do that. Keeping yourself engaged in physical activities that you find fun will help you stay active throughout your menopause journey. You don't have to go for something hard and painful; sticking to the activities you enjoy is always a much better option.

Here are some ideas to try:

- playing frisbee in the park
- attending a local gym
- going snowboarding with friends
- hosting a dance party
- holding swimming contests
- using stairs instead of the elevator

- going on a brisk walk every day

All these activities are not only fun to do, but will also make you sweat, burn those calories, and keep you energetic all day long!

Barriers Do Exist—Don't Let Them Stop You

Exercising is not always going to be easy. You might inevitably face some barriers while you try to incorporate healthy workouts into your routine. These barriers can be identified as internal or external. External barriers could be the environment, and the internal ones can be personal such as attitudes (Vermaak, n.d.). Let's take a look at a few barriers you might encounter and how to overcome them:

- **Family responsibilities:** If you have a baby or a younger child who needs to be tended to constantly, they could become a possible hurdle in your workout routine. You can ask your friends or neighbors to look after your children while you work out. If you can't leave your children at all, go out with them for a walk or stroll around the park. You can also try working out when they are sleeping or away at school.
- **Culture-specific expectations:** If you feel as if the people around you won't support you working out, try to explain to them that you want to work out for the sake of your physical and mental health. You can develop new friendships with people who are exercising, interact with them, and have your own workout buddies. That way, you'll feel accepted and have a group of your own to share your gym stories or workouts with.
- **Experiences of racism and issues with cultural or religious clothing:** If you have faced racism or have

people in your area who would have a problem with your culture and religious clothing, it's best to stick to places that accept you. If you don't have such places to go, stay at home and build a workout routine from the comfort of your home.

- **Money issues:** The cost of gym memberships or workout equipment can be restrictive for some. However, there are a lot of free or low-cost options, such as jogging, dancing, or cycling. You can use your resourcefulness and creativity and create DIY equipment as well.

- **Safety concerns:** If you don't feel comfortable exercising outdoors in your neighborhood, try some self-defense classes and explore local community resources that may offer affordable or free fitness programs.

- **Being overweight:** Don't let anyone tell you that going to work out isn't going to help because you are overweight. Don't push yourself to the point where you start feeling bad about yourself. Focus on the positives and realize that you have already taken the first step to shed that unwanted weight. Learn to reward yourself and pay no heed to rude comments. Listen to them from one ear, and throw them out the other.

INCORPORATING PHYSICAL ACTIVITY INTO EVERYDAY LIFE

Whether you love exercising or sticking to your sofa all day long, it's no surprise that moving and sitting less can have amazing effects on your body. However, adding a vigorous set of exercises may seem challenging.

If you are getting overwhelmed that you won't be able to do it, don't worry. You can always start small before jumping into the deep end. Here are some small ways you can increase your daily activity:

- **Take the stairs:** Make it a habit to take the stairs instead of the elevator throughout the day. If you feel as if you have been sitting for too long, then you can always climb a few flights.
- **Dance while you clean:** You can make those everyday chores a whole lot better if you add some dancing. Turn on your favorite beats that make you sway and then dance while you work. You'll burn calories and have fun!
- **Walk when you talk:** It's not always necessary to sit down while you take calls. Instead of staying glued to your seat, change things up a bit and walk while you talk. Some office spaces have even introduced the concept of walking paths to make it easier to burn while you earn.
- **Sit on exercise balls:** Sounds fun, right? Yes, it is. Sitting on a chair requires zero muscle activity. However, if you start sitting on those big exercise balls, you have to maintain your weight and balance, which is most likely to work your muscles. If you can't do that at work, start doing it while you're at home.

I get that starting a workout routine can be scary, confusing, and, honestly, just overwhelming. A lot of the time we're simply busy and don't understand where to fit in a demanding workout.

Start with these tips to get more movement into your daily, and then try scheduling workouts like you schedule your meetings, run to your errands instead of taking any sort of transportation, or get up early and do them first thing in the morning.

INCORPORATING A HEALTHY MINDSET

Here are some tips to help you generate a positive mindset while getting into your daily workout routine:

- **Focus on fun, health, and family enjoyment:** Get your family to take part in the physical exercises, too. Focus on the benefits everyone will enjoy, such as better sleep, good mood, and positive energy.
- **Reinforce what bodies can do, not how they look:** Don't focus on the bodily changes that can come with working out. Focus on how your self-esteem has improved or how confident you are. These factors matter most.
- **Keep your mindset around movement positive:** Remember, what you tell your brain is what it will believe. If you harbor negative comments such as, *I get so tired after exercising.* It won't be long before you get demotivated. Shift the narrative to the positive. Think of how energetic you feel after a workout routine.
- **Share feelings of reward and accomplishment out loud:** Along with daily affirmations, develop a habit of saying your compliments out loud. The more you hear them, the better you'll feel.

- **Build body confidence:** Building your physical endurance is going to make you feel good about yourself. It is the living proof of how far you have come in terms of training and hard work.
- **Avoid using exercise as punishment:** Ensure that your physical activity is something you look forward to, not something you use to torture yourself with. If you limit exercise only as a means of punishment, you'll never be able to enjoy it wholeheartedly.
- **Take baby steps:** Ensure that you take small steps toward your goals. Join an exercise club or find a gym partner to work out with, do what you enjoy, and make physical activity a part of your daily routine to stay motivated.

Working out is vital during menopause, and it can have major positive impacts on your life. Coming up with a routine that works for you can be tough but not impossible. Be flexible with your routines, have fun, and remember that working out has numerous benefits, including lifting your mood, improving your sleep, lowering risks of conditions that become risky during menopause, and improving your strength and stamina.

As we delve into Chapter 5, we'll now look at how creating social ties and having interactions is just as imperative as taking care of yourself mentally and physically during your transformative journey of menopause.

Help Others by Sharing Your Thoughts

"I was part of a cycle that desperately needed to be broken. There was a lack of open conversation and resources to help women navigate the changes we go through. That's why I'm now so passionate about raising awareness and encouraging more honest conversations." —Naomi Watts

Just like life is a canvas, menopause is like a bold and unpredictable brushstroke that can change a woman's life forever. It's something every woman experiences at some point in her life—a remarkable transition when monthly periods stop appearing after 12 months of perimenopause. Although the symptoms can linger for over a decade, it marks a significant shift from childbearing to non- childbearing years. It's a time of remarkable hormonal changes, typically occurring in the late 30s, 40s, or early 50s, bringing about not only biological but also emotional and physical adjustments. Our mission is to make [Conquering Menopause] accessible to everyone, to help women navigate this journey. To achieve this mission, we need your help in reaching everyone.

Would you extend a helping hand to someone you've never met, even without expecting credit for it?

This person we're talking about, she's a lot like you. Or at least, she used to be. She's seeking guidance, wanting to make a difference, but unsure where to start.

Your gift doesn't cost a dime and takes less than 60 seconds to give, but it can change a fellow reader's life forever. Your review could help...

...a small business provide for its community.

...an entrepreneur support their family.

...an employee find meaningful work.

...a client transform their life.

...a dream come true.

To make a real difference and experience that 'feel-good' moment, all you have to do is leave a review. Scan the QR code below to share your thoughts:

Your biggest fan, Samarra James.

PS - Fun fact: When you provide something of value to another person, it makes you more valuable to them. If you believe this book will help another woman, send it her way and watch the goodwill flow.

5

CONNECTIONS MATTER

Approximately 70% of women claim that menopause affects their marriages and their relationships in a negative way, proven by a survey conducted by The Family Law Menopause Project and Newson Health Research and Education in 2022. However, only a fifth of these women seek help to understand how to navigate this change (Urbanski, 2022).

There is a peak in divorce rates for women between the ages of 45 to 50 (Urbanski, 2022). The lack of awareness of this topic by the public results in many women questioning menopause as a cause of familial problems. According to a study, 86% of women are uncomfortable approaching the subject when it comes to professionals, and this takes a toll on their mental health when going through a divorce or separation process (Urbanski, 2022).

In this chapter, I will explain the intrinsic nature of menopause and how to prevent it from affecting our relationships with our partners, family, friends, and community.

IDENTIFYING THE PROBLEM

The first step to solving a problem is understanding its signs. Menopause brings about many physical and mental changes in our bodies, which can result in our bodies gaining weight, having low hormone levels, and experiencing mood swings, as discussed previously. These changes bring about the most difficulties when in a romantic relationship. Let's discuss how to keep your relationship from falling apart, as well as how to nurture it.

NURTURING THE PARTNER RELATIONSHIP

None of us want to have our relationships jeopardized due to uncontrollable body changes. We can protect the important relationships in our lives by addressing the problems we face. Here are some tips to help ensure you maintain a healthy and loving relationship with your partner:

- **Schedule a date night:** Something as simple as a couple's routine together or a weekly activity can do wonders for two people to grow closer as a pair. Allowing yourselves to take some time out of your schedule to spend with one another builds a healthy foundation for a loving and lasting relationship. Experiment by cooking together or taking part in morning and night routines.
- **Make sure to check in:** Allow yourself the time to ask your partner about their day, feelings, and worries. Developing trust and confidence in the bond between you is essential to lessen the effects menopause has on your mental health. Healthy communication deepens the connection between you and your partner by letting them feel that they have your attention. Also, provide them with

the opportunity to return the gesture. It's essential to find the balance between giving and taking.

- **Understand the importance of alone time:** It's okay to want to be alone in your personal space while in a relationship. With a positive understanding of personal space and boundaries, you can allow yourself to spend some time of your day doing whatever helps you to relax, such as reading or working out. The same applies to your partner. Some time, such as during meals, can be used to engage in conversations, allowing you to reconnect with your partner for the day with new experiences and stories to share.

- **Prioritize your relationship:** When going through the challenges of menopause, it is common to distract yourself by developing different hobbies or overworking. However, it is important to ponder your priorities and understand where your relationship with your partner stands. It is essential to make sure that your partner can feel your emotional, if not physical, contribution to your relationship. Take some time for them on a date out in the fresh air or a night indoors for just the two of you.

- **Talk about your problems:** Menopause creates a sense of vulnerability for a woman, and it is common to feel overwhelmed by it. In many cases, the thought of discussing the health issues created by menopause, including but not limited to the topic of sex, may cause women to feel embarrassed. It is vital to understand that our partners are incapable of understanding our desires and needs if we aren't able to voice them. So, talk about your problems with your partner so they can understand you and make you feel better.

- **Celebrate each other:** We often take even the smallest of moments for granted. However, we should take the opportunity to celebrate small milestones. Whether it is a few days free of pain medication or a decrease in the intensity of a mood swing, it's a good enough excuse to spend time with your significant other in happiness. Motivate each other to have a positive outlook. Menopause should not be a reason to hold yourself back from feeling alive.

- **Prioritize open communication:** Communication may sound easy, but when it comes down to trying to express how you feel to your partner without being able to give it a name, it becomes all the more difficult. It is one of the biggest reasons why we women hesitate when approaching the reason for our mood swings or turn away from the prospect of involving our significant others. This withdrawal must be addressed for the safety of our mental health. Never hesitate to approach your partner if only to help each other figure out your feelings by talking it out. Feelings don't necessarily have to be labeled to give you a sense of calm. Sometimes, knowing that someone you love understands your feelings and can help you navigate through them.

- **Learn about menopause together:** Communication is an important tool but it will reach an impasse if your partner is ill-informed of menopause and your needs as you experience it. It's important to understand and research about menopause. It never hurts to know about what you're going through rather than allowing yourself and your partner to experience changes without any clue.

- **Lean in to opportunities for intimacy:** Is intimacy synonymous with sex? Is it possible to be intimate without it turning into something sexual? Intimacy does not require you to force yourself through complex emotions to feel sexually charged for your partner. It is alright to withdraw from the thought of sex when going through menopause while simultaneously craving intimacy. Just a close snuggling session with your partner or the close warmth of their body while doing a hobby, such as pottery together, is enough to maintain the level of intimacy. Don't fear your partner's disappointment. If the communication is strong, they will understand how you need to feel close.

- **Embrace a shared active lifestyle:** Work out, walk in the fresh air, jog to the park, or learn new dances to impress others at parties. Encourage your body to move and remain active while spending quality time with your significant other by having them be your workout buddy. Hype each other up and have friendly competitions. They aren't only your lover, they can be your best friend, too.

- **Draw on patience and understanding:** It is vital to have these two qualities both for you and your partner. Your partner should be able to give you space and time should you require it when facing the negative aspects of menopause. However, our responsibility is also to be patient and understanding with our partners as they learn to adapt to our needs. No one is born prepared for the effects of menopause, but we can learn to adapt together.

- **Address finances:** While maintaining your relationship is important, we must look into the practical aspects such as calculating finances for the medical requirements that come with the onset of menopause. Medical expenses can be brought up in a conversation so you can involve your partner and discuss how to tackle financial contributions.

- **Enlist the support of experts:** It is not shameful to admit that not everything can be solved with only our partner by our side. Sometimes, a third person needs to mediate conversations and guide us through effective tools that may have not occurred to us before.

- **Support your individuality:** Is my happiness reliant on my partner's contribution as I go through menopause? Self-reflection and meditation are essential to ensure that you feel satisfied with your growth and navigate through the journey of menopause without being too dependent on your partner. They provide welcomed companionship, but it is important to maintain a sense of individuality. Allow yourself to embrace this new opportunity on your terms and enjoy the positive sides while also powering through the negative sides.

- **Focus on the positives:** Positivity is key both for you and your partner. Look for the silver lining when faced with thunderous clouds and enjoy the rain. Hold your partner by the hand and dance with smiles on your faces. There may be some days when it gets too much and smiling seems impossible. However, a simple hand interlocked with another is enough.

The Difference Between Loneliness and Being Alone

Many women go through loss as a lover departs from this world and some face menopause alone. One interviewer talked to a couple's counselor who gave insight into the difference between loneliness and being alone: "One way that I help individuals process the loss of a partner is to help them reframe their feelings of 'loneliness' into 'being alone.' I do not recommend moving on to another relationship until you are comfortable being alone. Once you are, you're much less likely to attract the wrong person into your life" (Dolgen, 2017).

Finding comfort in ourselves will guide us to be the best version of ourselves. Allow love to find you once more, in whatever form it takes.

WHAT DO WE DO IF WE ARE BOTH IN MENOPAUSE?

Both you and your partner don't need to go through the same symptoms at the same time while in menopause. The symptoms and resulting emotional and physical changes vary from person to person. Where one might require intimacy, the other may want more space. Having menopause simultaneously doesn't always lead to understanding from both sides.

One Couple's Journey

One article stated that due to the increase in patients undergoing gender confirmation surgeries, there will be many people part of the LGBTQ+ community who will be experiencing menopause in the future (Sutton, 2021). So, how can you navigate through menopause when your partner is going through the same thing?

Let's take an example from an experience shared by a lesbian couple. Menopause reared its head in what seemed like an instant, causing a disturbance in Taz and Asha's peaceful lives.

Asha was the first to experience the effects of her menopause with uncontrollable bursts of anger and irritation. However, these attacks were unintentional, resulting in both women crumbling under the emotional struggle of understanding these new negative emotions. However, with trust and perseverance, they created the safe word rule that would allow them to communicate through their bubbling emotions with only a simple word. Soon after, Taz suffered menopause symptoms as well, her emotions favoring anxiety and panic.

Taz's treatment needed more than safe words; she needed a medical professional. Even as two women in a relationship together, menopause put their relationship to the test. Neither needed the same treatment to ease their troubles, but by realizing their relationship was worth fighting for and knowing the importance of medical help, they overcame a difficult time in their lives (Foster, 2022).

Understanding Your Unique Relationship

Following Asha and Taz's example, the first step is to understand how menopause affects you and your partner. For some, it is through uncontrolled outbursts, and for others, it's anxiety and depression. You must also observe how your menopause is affecting your partner. Is there a mutual understanding of your health or are either of you confused by the sudden change in behavior?

The last thing we want to do is hurt those we love. To prevent that, we must remain well informed of our health as well as theirs. Some couples opt to go for HRT treatment to lower the effects of menopause while others manage to pull through successfully.

There may be moments when the relationship is strained through arguments and clashing opinions. If this happens, it is best to seek professional help if the matter seems out of control.

Another important point to consider is that women are not the only people who go through menopause. Trans men are assigned the female gender at birth and people who identify as non-binary go through menopause as well and enter the realm of gender dysmorphia. Being forced to acknowledge the existence of female hormones in the body while not identifying as that gender creates discomfort and reluctance to seek help from medical professionals.

The problems don't just lie there either. There is a lack of knowledge about healthcare and trans awareness, resulting in people opting out of having themselves checked entirely. The worst thing to hear while also suffering from emotional turmoil is to feel unrecognized as your true identity by being misgendered. Inclusivity is important as basic respect and understanding for the multiple patients who walk into a clinic with hopes of easing their pain.

For example, Sam is a trans-man who feels anxiety and discomfort when having to face medical issues labeled as part of female healthcare. "I'm forced to confront the fact that my body doesn't naturally produce testosterone, but it does produce estrogen. I experience a lot of dysphoria about that," he said (Sutton, 2021). Words play an important impact in making or breaking someone's self-esteem. No one wants to be excluded or invalidated. Forcing trans people to question their reality and their health is cruel.

While learning how to navigate through menopause, allow yourself to be an advocate for other people as well. Use words that allow people who go through this change to feel included and seen. We should help each other and motivate one another to overcome. We may not have the same symptoms; however, it affects all of us no matter how we identify ourselves. Open your hearts to empathy and companionship so we can make this time easier for ourselves and others.

REKINDLING INTIMACY

Menopause often makes us feel undesirable. It's tough to love your body or even think about initiating intimacy when your body aches and your head feels like it is out to get you. I imagine we don't have the best words to describe ourselves when we are at our lowest. Sometimes, it's not about what's in our heads but the decrease in sexual needs.

However, intimacy and sexual interactions are important to make a relationship feel alive. Override the voice in your head that speaks against you because it's lying to you. Motivate yourself to pursue romance and prove to yourself that you can still enjoy sex in new ways. Here are some tips to guide you:

- **Think about sex:** If your brain tells you no, take control and demand yes. You control your thoughts, and no matter how difficult it may seem, you can take control again. Allow yourself to think about sex with your partner. Recall the warmth, the gentle touches, and the fluttering in your chest as you felt the build-up exciting you. There is no harm in fantasizing and imagining while listening to erotica. Who knows? Maybe it'll give you some ideas for the future!

- **Make an intimate appointment:** Try creating a calendar for sex. Each day can bring a new experience or something fun to try. As we age and our lives get more entangled with work and busy schedules, sometimes it's best to have good old-fashioned planned encounters.

- **Change course from intercourse:** Perhaps the usual isn't working out for you. Not a problem because there are always new things to try! There are long baths together with fancy products and scents, deep hugs in bed with only the warmth of another body to focus on, rediscovering your body with or without a partner to see where new sensitivities lie, and other creative ways to feel pleasure.

- **Shop for sex:** Don't be shy to shop when it comes to fun in the bedroom. Sometimes, we try everything we can but lack the excitement a new toy brings. Creams, lubricants, oils, clothes, and toys can turn up the temperature. However, make sure your safety is also a priority. It is essential to check for allergic reactions and personal preferences when it comes to both you and your partner.

- **Focus on your body — inside and out:** Love your body and cherish it with new vigor by eating healthy, enjoying the outdoors, and sleeping on a maintained schedule. When our love for our bodies grows, we look forward to expressing it. Your worth should not be dictated by the opinions of others. Rather, it should stem from your positive thinking.

- **Speak up:** Improving your sexual desires should not come with the cost of your comfort. Sometimes, it's not new and creative ways of sex that you need but rather the attention of a healthcare professional. One article states: "Some women experience vaginal dryness or vaginal atrophy with a decrease in estrogen that can make intercourse less enjoyable or painful. Others may have more difficulty sensing stimulation. Hot flashes, night sweats, and insomnia take their toll on energy levels, causing fatigue. Medications, too, can dull libido" (WHN Editorial Team, 2022). Discover the options around you that provide you the most comfort and safety, whether it comes in the form of long talks with your partner or therapy by a sex counselor. Have a conversation with your beloved by using "I" statements, directing the conversation toward your fears, emotions, and wants while in menopause. Don't be scared to ask for something and see if your partner is comfortable with that. Intimacy is not worth it if both of you aren't enjoying being close to each other.

- **Don't stop:** Age shouldn't stop you from enjoying something that provides you with comfort and pleasure. There is no shame in experiencing one of the best parts of life at your age. Why follow a toxic society that forces you to believe that youth is ideal to feel beautiful? Besides, with more sex, there is always the advantage of better and more satisfying experiences in the future. Enjoy your body while embracing the change and experiencing new forms of pleasure with your partner.

Birth Control Tips/Contraceptives and Menopause

An important factor of intimacy to consider is the probability of conception and the safe use of contraceptives while in menopause. The fertility rate drops as you reach the age of 30, but unplanned pregnancies are still possible if you're not taking appropriate measures, especially during the premenopausal phase. Some advisable contraceptives during this time include:

- Hormonal oral pills reduce ovulation, thicken cervical mucus, and thin out the uterus lining to prevent pregnancy.
- Non-oral hormonal birth control comes in the form of vaginal rings, skin patches, or shots.
- Intrauterine devices (IUDs) are placed by a doctor in the uterus through the vagina.
- Barrier methods include female and male condoms, spermicides, cervical caps, or spermicide sponges. Keep in mind that these methods are not the best at contraception.
- Sterilization is a permanent solution for contraception.
- Emergency birth control or "morning after pills" are orally taken as a backup in case your choice of birth control fails. These are taken between 72 hours to 5 days after intercourse depending on the type of pill.

Note that every choice of contraception must be discussed with your doctor to prevent aggravating your body or threatening your health with possible side effects.

Menopausal patients should rely less on contraceptive pills and more on condoms and contraceptive surgery when reaching their 40s. Where there is still a possibility of conceiving after the mid-40 or 50 years, pills, though very effective, may cause blood clots, high blood pressure, and other health problems. Not everyone faces the same health issues, but it's better to be safe than sorry.

Oral contraceptive pills can numb the pain caused by premenopause, but it is not recommended due to the possibility of health issues. Hormone therapy is a safer option with each session adjusted to your body's needs.

With all this information and tips, you're well-equipped to tackle your relationship with your partner and renew love, trust, and intimacy with nothing holding you back. We must push forward with determination, knowing that we will not allow society to shape us or invalidate our bodies when we can love and treasure them.

ENGAGING FAMILY AND FRIENDS

Familial relationships and our friendships hold a lot of importance in our lives. It's why their contribution to our comfort, under-standing, and relief affects us so much. We go through many phys-ical, emotional, and spiritual changes in menopause, but did you know that your family's support can make a big difference for you? Family support during menopause eases its symptoms and helps you avoid spiraling into loneliness and isolation. Here are some ways you can gain the support of your support system:

- **Get educated about menopause:** You can only inform your family about your health if you are well-informed yourself. Discuss your symptoms and conditions with your doctor and spend time researching menopause and its symptoms even if you haven't experienced them yet. After you have collected all your information, sit down with your friends and family to educate them about the changes occurring in your body and how you're hoping to navigate through it with their help. Help them understand that you require their support, reassurance, and assistance in your everyday life.

- **Think about how your symptoms may impact others:** Unchecked emotions expressed in random outbursts can hurt people even when you don't intend to. However, hurting them by accident does not excuse the fact that they were hurt without having any information about your condition. Only by knowing the true extent of your pain can they practice patience and understanding around you. They can become a source of laughter when you're feeling down and a warm hug when you need one.

- **Understand that honesty is the best policy:** Avoid vague answers to questions about your well-being. Doing so will only confuse those around you and worsen your mood due to the lack of understanding. Talk things out or create a system where you can communicate your emotions with fewer words when it becomes too overwhelming for you to hold a conversation. Communication with your partner is important when it comes to your opinion and your body's reaction to sex. Do not let your body hurt by forcing it through sexual acts that should be "normal." Listen to your body and communicate its message to your partner so they can understand as well.

- **Talk about what you're going through:** Menopause is not a taboo subject. People with a uterus and female hormones will go through this change. It's important to not consider it as a disease of shameful sickness either. Be transparent with your family and involve them with your emotions and physical pain. Talking to older people who have gone through similar experiences will provide you with more insight.

- **Ask for help:** Don't apologize when your body is changing in its natural way. Don't fear asking for help, just as you wouldn't if you had a physical injury.

MENOPAUSE AT WORK

It is sometimes scary to think that menopause is capable of creating symptoms so powerful that they can affect your work attendance, performance, and career development. Some of the effects include exhaustion, insomnia, weak memory, and poor concentration (O'Neill et al., 2023).

Considering that this is a medical development experienced by many people, we should learn how to cope with this change and have our place of work adapted to fit certain requirements. The number of people going through menopause in the workplace is increasing, so it is imperative to involve this topic as a part of office discussions.

However, there are a few people who do not wish to involve their workspace with their health and opt for managing their menopausal symptoms instead. Here are some tips for creating a healthy lifestyle that will help you continue to succeed in the workplace:

- **Go to bed early:** Approximately eight to nine hours of sleep is optimal for a healthy working body. Prioritize having a regular sleeping schedule every day so your body can have its required rest for the busy day ahead.
- **Drink plenty of water:** Hydration is a must when going through the stress and hot flashes that burden your body.

An average of eight glasses of water a day is mandatory. You can also bring in a portable fan to cool you off at the office.

- **Dress in layers:** Dressing in multiple layers gives you the option of removing them as you find comfortable during a hot flash. Make sure to keep that office fan near you to control your body temperature.
- **Watch your diet:** Caffeine, alcohol, and spicy foods are a big no if you want to avoid the worst effects of your symptoms. Invest in a diet packed with calcium, vitamin D, whole grains, and vegetables.
- **Take a walk:** Try to fit in some exercise during your office lunch breaks. No need to hit the gym—a few miles will adjust your body to a healthy body weight and sleep schedule and lessen the severity of menopause pain, making you a happier person.
- **Quit smoking:** Smoking is a habit that will put you at risk for early menopause, intensifying painful symptoms, and contributing to sleepless nights and anxiety, It's best to stop while you can and save your body from that pain.
- **Stay on top of organization:** Organize your work with less multi-tasking to avoid straining your mind and focus on completing work efficiently.
- **Talk to a friend:** Talk to co-workers about your issues rather than staying silent and treating the topic as taboo. Find other women going through the same experience and create a support group to help each other.
- **Don't be afraid to seek medical help:** Never downplay your pain and force yourselves to work while suffering. When things get too difficult, consult your doctor for a check-up and perhaps even get their opinion on hormone replacement therapy or other treatments to ease your pain.

Communication With Employers About Menopause

When experiencing menopausal symptoms, it is always best to communicate with your employer about it so they can provide you with flexibility and adjusted hours wherever possible. Many hesitate to approach the topic of menopause because it is considered a private topic. However, know that it is your right to take control and express concerns for your health. If you wish for your discussion to remain confidential, book an appointment with a Human Resources representative.

Communicate with full transparency how menopause is affecting your work, what your contribution is to controlling these effects, and how your employer can help you during this time. It is imperative that your employer understands where you're coming from and knows that discrimination based on gender is against the law. Know your rights and try to make your workspace a place of comfort.

A Healthy Work-Life Balance

For some people, there is a thin line between work and home life. For people going through menopause, it is essential to keep that line in mind and prioritize health before work. There is no use in working yourself to the bone if you aren't able to enjoy the success that comes with it. If we keep on focusing on the minute details and blowing them out of proportion in panic, we'll lose ourselves in workload and menopausal pain. It's important to step back and see the whole picture to remind ourselves why we are here. Dr. Ghazala Aziz-Scott says, "Many larger corporations already have policies in place that offer support for employees going through menopause" (*Menopause in the Workplace*, 2022).

This should be motivation to voice your concerns about your health with coworkers and employers. If your current career path seems like too much of a burden, perhaps it's time to search for an alternate path that'll provide you with satisfaction and ease. Work shouldn't have to be accepted as a struggle, it can be a source of happiness, too.

EMBRACING COMMUNITY SUPPORT DURING MENOPAUSE

Psychotherapist Esther Perel is known for saying, "The quality of our relationships determines the quality of our lives" (*The Health Benefits of Social Support During the Menopausal Transition*, n.d.). However, menopause can cause a person to isolate themselves. Often, we feel as if we cannot communicate with anybody about something so private and that it's something we should control to not burden anyone else.

However, the truth is that there are support groups in the community that are more than willing to share experiences and offer aid where needed in person and online. If there is no such support group near you, take the first step to form one and help others in your neighborhood with similar experiences. We can reclaim our identities and positive outlook on life by enjoying each other's company on walks, picnics, and even a fancy brunch. Everyone knows we deserve it!

Menopause may try to convince us that the only way we can get through it is if we do it alone. However, our interactions with others and the love we receive from our friends and family are truly the best ways to make this change bearable. Who says we must suffer in silence?

We should be proud of the people we have connections with and trust them to support us in our time of need. With our shared experiences, we can help each other and take the first steps to making important decisions regarding our health. It is not just you against the world—it is all of us working together.

Let's move on to the next chapter, where we'll explore various treatment options for menopause and help you determine what is right for you. From hormonal treatment options to natural remedies, there are many medical and holistic options available, so you don't have to suffer in silence!

6

EMPOWERED CHOICES

Across the globe, 73% of women reported that they were not doing anything to treat their menopause symptoms. Moreover, in a survey based in the United States by The State of Menopause Study, it was found that 29% of women had never taken an interest in researching menopause before they experienced it. Where 20% of women suffer from menopausal symptoms for over a year before meeting a medical professional, 34% continue life without being properly diagnosed (Gordon, 2021).

That alarming statistic makes it clear that women, whether they have started their periods or are near menopause, should continuously be assessed and equipped with resources to make well-informed decisions. It is highly unfortunate that although all women experience menopause, very few acknowledge it due to the stigma around it.

In this chapter, we'll delve into the treatment options available to manage and embrace menopause, along with stress management and proactive healthy advocacy to ensure that women around the globe feel comfortable enough to embrace their menopause with convenience, ease, and without fear of judgment.

EXPLORING TREATMENT OPTIONS FOR MENOPAUSE

There is a wide range of treatment options available for women dealing with menopause, both conventional and alternative therapies. Some of them are:

- **Hormone replacement therapy (HRT):** Menopause results in low levels of estrogen, which increases the risks of bone loss among other problems. By starting a low dose of estrogen around the time of menopause, as per your doctor's instructions, you can lower these risks and also relieve yourself from intense hot flashes. For those without a uterus, they must take estrogen as well as progesterone. However, long-term use of this treatment can lead to cardiovascular and breast cancer.
- **Vaginal estrogen:** Vaginal dryness is a common symptom of menopause that can be treated by estrogen creams, rings, or tablets for estrogen to be absorbed by the vaginal tissue. This will bring comfort during intercourse and relieve urinary problems.
- **Low-dose antidepressants:** Women who can't take estrogen due to medical reasons are provided a low dose of antidepressants, classed as selective serotonin reuptake inhibitors (SSRIs) to treat hot flashes.
- **Gabapentin (Gralise, Horizant, Neurontin):** An alternate treatment to estrogen therapy is Gabaepentin, which is used for seizures but can also aid with nightly hot flashes.
- **Clonidine (Catapres, Kapvay):** Clonidine is often used to treat hypertension and can also be used as an alternative for hot flashes.

- **Cognitive behavioral therapy:** Cognitive behavioral therapy, or CBT, allows you to talk to a professional about your experience with menopause. This method of therapy aids with anxiety and depression while also providing a safe space to overcome the vulnerability of talking about menopause.

Regardless of the treatments listed, it's always best to consult your doctor before making any decision to determine the balance of benefits and risks.

HORMONAL TREATMENTS: PROS AND CONS

Hormonal treatments (HTs) are a commonly preferred solution for menopausal symptoms to increase hormone levels our bodies aren't able to produce anymore. Estrogen therapy provides estrogen to the body, preferably in low doses by a doctor. Estrogen progesterone/progestin hormone therapy (EPT) is a combination treatment providing both estrogen and progesterone. However, as much as hormone treatments are capable of easing us through the most painful symptoms of menopause, it is vital to be aware of the risks that can come with its use as well.

Benefits of Hormone Treatment

With hormone treatment, night sweats, hot flashes, itchy skin, and vaginal dryness are no longer a cause of great concern. This treatment is proven to prevent osteoporosis and decrease the probability of fractures. In an article for Cedars Sinai, Koren Wetmore (2023) states:

"A study of more than 25,000 postmenopausal women aged 50–79 found that hormone therapy reduced the risk of fractures. This is especially important for those whose uterus and ovaries were removed before age 45. Women who experience this "surgical menopause" have a higher risk of bone loss and osteoporosis."

Another point of concern is how, during menopause, our bodies attempt to produce energy from the fats in our brain's white matter, putting us at risk of Alzheimer's. We can reduce the risk if we start hormone treatment before menopause; however, this benefit no longer takes effect once menopause is underway. In that case, a ketogenic diet is a good preventive method. This treatment allows us to improve our lifestyle and mood once the mental and physical effects of menopause no longer have a hold on us. Moreover, it lowers the risk of tooth loss, colon cancer, and diabetes.

Risks of Hormone Treatment

Hormone treatments are not without their risks. With long-term use, they increase the risk of breast cancer and blood clots, as well as gallbladder or gallstone problems. Patients who still have a uterus must receive combination (estrogen and progesterone) treatment to prevent the possibility of uterine cancer. It's hard to believe that a treatment that if started before midlife can prevent dementia and Alzheimer's is the same treatment that can increase the risk of it if started after midlife.

Everyone who experiences menopause is unique in body type, needs, and experiences. We cannot say for sure which treatment will work for whom. Your doctor, with detailed information on your medical history, can guide you in the right direction. However, there are a few key factors to look out for when considering hormone treatments. Do not consider hormone treatment if:

- you have suffered from breast or endometrial cancer.
- you have abnormal vaginal bleeding.

- you have suffered from blood clots or your body remains at high risk.
- you have suffered from heart attacks or stroke or are at risk of vascular diseases.
- you are pregnant. (It's important to get tested just in case.)
- you have liver disease.

If you decide to consult your doctor to receive hormone therapy, it's better to keep its side effects in mind. Most commonly, people experience monthly bleeding along with random spotting, breast tenderness, and mood swings. Some unusual side effects include fluid retention, headaches, skin discolorations, increased breast density, and itchiness under estrogen patches.

Knowledge is power and this is indeed the case wherever your body is concerned. Ensure that you are well informed of all your choices, including their pros and cons, before making any decision regarding your health. Your body is your responsibility, and it's up to you to take care of it.

BIOHACKING SOLUTIONS FOR MENOPAUSE

There are many ways to help reduce the effects of menopause, and biohacking is one of them. Biohacking solutions are alternate methods to hormone treatments. They are the practice of methods applied from different fields such as biology, genetics, neuroscience, and nutrition to enhance physical or mental health for a specific goal. Kimberly Dawn Neumann (2023) quotes author Dave Asprey in her article:

"[Biohacking] is a global movement based on the idea that you can change the environment around you and inside of you so you have full control of your biology."

You can look into multiple different biohacking solutions to find an ideal solution for you:

Red Light Therapy

We are now aware of menopause and what changes it brings to our bodies. Exactly what is red light therapy and how does it help with menopause? Invented by NASA to mimic the sun's most beneficial wavelengths and recreate red and near-infrared light, this treatment uses this light to penetrate the body at different depths. At a cellular level, it promotes energy production and boosts cellular health. By penetrating the skin, it allows increased production of elastin and collagen for youthful skin. By stimulating the release of nitric oxide in our blood, it aids in improving cardiovascular and kidney health. Not to mention the improved mood after the therapy as beta-endorphins are released.

The effects of genitourinary syndrome, such as low libido, UTIs, less natural lubrication, and itching, can be improved by hormone regulation and circulation through red light therapy. No longer will we have to shuffle around uncomfortably in public or at home. Our skin becomes one of the targets of menopause, which also has hopes of being treated through red light therapy due to its anti-inflammatory and immunity-boosting abilities. Improved blood levels and hair growth are a result of red light therapy working its magic through science.

Not to mention, red light therapy aids with more complex issues as well. For example, thyroid problems and menopause are never a good combination. They have similar symptoms, and if a person with thyroid imbalances reaches menopause, their symptoms get worse. Luckily, with the red light treatment, your thyroid hormones will be regulated easily. One article states, "According to the Sleep Foundation, 39% to 47% of perimenopausal women and a whopping 35% to 60% of postmenopausal women experience trouble falling or staying asleep, which can also negatively impact their physical health and cognitive function" (Garcia, 2023).

The near-infrared (NIR) and red light used in this therapy are the same wavelengths that encourage your body to rest, an easy solution to sleepless nights. Hot flashes are suspected to be due to the hypersensitivity of your hypothalamus, which regulates body temperature. Red light therapy's contribution to hormone health optimization reduces the occurrence of these symptoms. The best part of this entire process is that there are no side effects!

Infrared Sauna Therapy

We read the word "sauna" and we're already excited. Luckily for us sauna lovers, a good steaming session is just what we need to ease our symptoms. A hot water bottle sure seems useless when compared to full-body relaxation. Infrared saunas can boost estrogen and vital protein production to reduce harsh hot flashes and relax your muscles and joints. Excessive sweating pushes extra water out from your body to combat fluid retention.

Similar to red light therapy, the wavelengths promote sleep and stimulate endorphin release to boost your mood. Other than reviving your skin and removing toxins from your body, this miracle sauna therapy reduces the risk of cardiovascular problems as well. I may have an idea of what's on our schedules now!

PEMF

PEMF stands for pulsed electromagnetic fields. It is an option to consider when thinking about your health while in menopause. PEMF therapy has a variety of benefits with its positive effects against menopausal symptoms. For example, we are already aware that low estrogen levels contribute to a high risk of fractures and low bone health. PEMF strengthens the bones, including teeth, to fight against this risk. It is also beneficial for muscle and joint pain, and due to its anti-inflammatory properties, it helps in maintaining the digestive system and relieves the skin. Not to mention the brain stimulation through this therapy reduces, headaches, bad moods, and hits of depression. Let's take a personal experience as an example:

"For the next 30 minutes, I just enjoyed and relaxed listening to the music. At the end of the treatment, I felt relaxed and chilled. A niggling backache had subsided, and I was breathing easier despite my cold" (*The 34 Symptoms of Menopause, PEMF Therapy Helps,* 2021).

I hope this gives an insight into what PEMF entails. Of course, a doctor's consultation is always important.

Vibration Therapy

Another biohacking technique to consider is vibration therapy, which promotes the improvement of health through biomechanical stimulation in the body by vibrations at various frequencies. Its ability to increase bone mass makes it a good treatment for osteoporosis among other conditions.

The human body is capable of sensing vibrations within a certain range, and this treatment is adjusted to keep that range in mind to ensure safety while in use. One article states, "Worldwide, annually, about 8.9 million fractures occur, most of which are due to osteopenia and osteoporosis" (Singh & Varma, 2023). Osteoporosis is a common threat for people experiencing menopause caused by estrogen deficiency, the risks of which increase as the body grows older. Along with fractures, it also affects our posture and joints and, in turn, worsens our physical activity and mood.

Having a corporate lifestyle forces less physical movement if work is confined to a desk and even less sunlight, which is important for vitamin D. So, vibration therapy is considered for those who are physically restricted. Supported by other pharmacological treatments, this method strengthens the muscles and bones after careful analysis of the body's requirements. The vibrations also improve blood circulation for better nutrition to the bones. Overall, it's a safe treatment that still requires research to improve its functionality further but is a great solution for those with physical restraints regarding movement.

Neurofeedback Training

Many prefer training their brain to ease their menopausal worries in comparison to other medical treatments. The first step is to look beyond the myth that this treatment confirms all the pain felt is superficial. This is never the case when it comes to menopause. Uterine and ovary functioning are believed to originate from the brain, so its dysregulation can create problems in their function as well.

Neurofeedback training affects many parts of your brain that help you regain control of your body. For example, the hypothalamus is affected to maintain body temperature, the hippocampus for memory, and the prefrontal cortex for concentration. It should be no surprise that a healthy brain aids in curing insomnia, rage, seizures, mood swings, and panic. It is a safe intervention with no need for medication.

NATURAL REMEDIES

We need to understand that depending on medical treatments and biohacking methods can't be the only solution for menopausal symptoms. We should try our best to improve our lifestyle for our bodies to improve.

For example, the first step should be to improve our diet by including vegetables, soy, calcium, lean protein, flaxseed, vitamin E, and vitamin D to improve our bones, weight, and muscles and relieve our hot flashes.

Make sure to avoid any trigger foods or spicy foods. In addition, it is best to refrain from drinks that cause dehydration and contain caffeine and alcohol. Fruit juices and water are healthier alternatives.

Moreover, our bodies need to remain in motion. Encourage yourself to exercise or practice yoga for a healthy mind and body. One article stated, "A study in Korea that looked at the effects of a 12-week walking exercise program found that the exercise improved physical and mental health and overall quality of life in a group of 40 menopausal women" (Stanten, 2021).

With a good diet, hydration, and exercise in mind, try to maintain an ideal body weight unless you are intermittent fasting. Your body requires energy for its functioning, and forcing your body to work without giving it sustenance is not a good idea. One other suggested method is to do what you believe is benefiting you as long as it doesn't worsen your condition. After all, your mind is powerful, and perhaps believing in your betterment will help you improve your mood.

If a massage or acupuncture does the trick, help yourself and enjoy a relaxing time. Although their effectiveness is unconfirmed, natural supplements are an option as long as you make sure to receive them from reputable sources and read the ingredients carefully. Be especially careful with supplements that claim to be a cure, as menopause is not a disease with a permanent solution. These may not be a permanent solution, but a lifestyle change can bring some relief.

MASTERING STRESS-MANAGEMENT TECHNIQUES

Preparing for menopause or going through menopause while researching ways to make it easier on yourself can be very stressful. But believe it or not, even if stressing about it seems like the best way to cope, it will only make things harder on you. It's natural to worry at times, but now that we know what we are dealing with, let's go through some ways we can manage our stress and avoid spiraling into even worse symptoms:

- **Mindfulness:** Sometimes, thinking about 10 things at once forces us to deviate from the present. We must focus on the now, and through exercises such as deep breathing and the five senses game, we can calm our minds to bring us back to the present and look at things a little more clearly and with more self-awareness. Take it one step at a time.
- **Meditation:** Oftentimes, we believe that sitting quietly with our eyes closed will do nothing more than waste our time. However, meditation is more than just the positioning of our bodies; it is an escape for our minds from all the troubles that cloud our thoughts. Allow yourself some relaxation with meditation and ease into the habit of spending some time every day. The difference in your mind will surprise you. I meditate in the morning in front of a window, so I can soak up the natural light the sunrise provides, easing me into my day.

- **Relaxation exercises:** During menopause, you become all too aware of your body getting stiff and painful. Keep your body in motion like a well-oiled machine by exercising or even enjoying slow yoga, such as Hatha yoga, to ease the mind and the physical body. Not to mention, with good exercise, a peaceful sleep at night lies ahead, which helps you remain stress-free, too.

- **Stress-reducing activities:** Things making you more stressed are a no-go. Instead, spend time with your friends and loved ones as a welcome distraction. If you would rather have some alone time, do what distracts you from your current state, such as reading a good book, revisiting well-loved hobbies, or learning new ones. Your comfort and happiness matter.

- **Balanced nutrition:** By following the previously mentioned tips regarding diets for menopausal women, you can ensure to remain stress-free without the fear of unhealthy weight gain and restless nights. Coffee and alcohol should never be your go-to stress relievers. Instead, enjoy making and eating food you know will make you happier and healthier.

- **Regular physical activity:** If workouts are not your thing, try to find physical activity benefits in other things. Explore the possibilities of passions in other sports such as swimming and even dancing. The more you try, the more your body will help by releasing endorphins to keep your mood alleviated. Walking is the easiest exercise you can do.

- **Supportive social connections:** Whether it be your partner, a friend, a menopause counselor, or a support group, allow yourself to break through that vulnerability and share your experiences. If that is too difficult as a first step, talk about anything a everything. Have meaningful conversations that make you laugh and smile. Feel good while being surrounded by people who you know, love you, and support you through this time.

- **Professional guidance:** Know that you're not alone in this battle. If planning your treatments, possible medication, and navigating through your personal life becomes too difficult, seek help from a professional who can guide you through your troubles with a properly structured approach. Sometimes, all we need is a secondary opinion of our problem to help us address it.

- **Positive affirmations:** There are times when our minds are cruel to us and hit us with negative thoughts about ourselves. Those thoughts follow us for a long time, and everything around us reminds us of them, sending us into a turmoil of self-doubt among other things. What we need to do to fight against this is to prove to ourselves that we are capable of loving ourselves as we are. The more your mind is filled with positive thoughts about yourself, the less space there is for negativity to reside. Why not look in the mirror and start with a smile for yourself? The second step can perhaps be a simple complement.

Yoga, Meditation, and Deep Breathing Exercises

There are many different ways to ensure your stress levels remain low. However, ways that require movement and participation of your mind and body allow you to feel a more conscious change. Let's discover the different techniques of yoga, meditation, and deep-breathing exercises.

Bryan D. Vargo gives a thorough tutorial on relaxation and deep breathing led by a registered yoga therapist, Stephanie Moonaz. The practice for deep breathing she suggests is to sit someplace with support to straighten your back. Shoulders must be shifted back and down, straightening your spine while keeping your ribs, sternum, and face relaxed. You must close your eyes with one hand on the abdomen and feel how each inhale pushes your abdomen toward the hand while each exhale draws you away from it. Spending a few minutes breathing like this and extending your breaths makes you aware of your body's movements.

For relaxing the body, she suggests lying on your back in a dark and quiet space with a blanket over the body; having your legs elevated is optional. You must first force all the muscles in your body to contract then slowly relax and feel the difference. After repeating this, it's best to slowly get a feel of your body before continuing with your day (Vargo, n.d.).

The active yogic breath, however, can be applied while walking as you try to fit in 10 steps between every inhale and exhale. You can always discover more techniques as you research what fits right for you.

Navigating through life is difficult for a lot of us, and every day brings a new struggle. It's worse when menopause causes even the smallest problems to seem so much more difficult to tackle. We need to be prepared to make sure that we don't succumb to the pressure and instead succeed through this difficult point in life by taking steps to remain stress-free and make the correct decisions.

REMOVING TOXINS FROM YOUR HOME AND PRODUCTS

According to a study, a woman whose body has a higher content of chemicals found in common items and self-care products is more likely to experience early menopause than a woman with a lower level of the same chemicals (*Earlier Menopause Linked to Everyday Chemical Exposures*, 2015). Another article states,

"Chemicals linked to earlier menopause may lead to an early decline in ovarian function, and our results suggest we as a society should be concerned," said senior author Amber Cooper, MD, an assistant professor of obstetrics and gynecology (Schmidt, 2017).

It was discovered that people with a healthier lifestyle undergo menopause at a later age compared to those with an unhealthy one. Ethnicities and nationalities also make a difference. However, the effects of the harmful chemicals around us play a great role, as they are considered endocrine-disrupting compounds that increase health risks (Schmidt, 2017). It is vital to be aware of this fact and see what we can do to prevent these chemicals from affecting us as best as we can.

A Guide to a Chemical-free Home

Even household items must be handled responsibly when they contain chemicals or biohazard symbols on the packaging. We must be well versed in the symbols we identify and use, store, and dispose of the products as described in their packaging. Try to keep your house chemical-free by making your cleaning supplies or finding chemical-free alternatives. Be careful when in the kitchen to use less plastic and prevent using high flame on non-stick cookware.

When shopping for cosmetics, it is always safe to be aware of the harmful chemicals that are added and to check the ingredients before purchase. Watch out for chemicals such as parabens, diethanolamine, or even fragrance ingredients.

It's always best to keep these chemicals labeled and away from children to avoid misuse. Keep contacts ready in case there is a medical emergency caused by these chemicals. We can't do anything about the chemicals in the air and soil, but we should try to do what's possible within our homes.

Another way to keep your home chemical-free is to look for eco-friendly substitutes online or to make some yourself. For example, who knew vinegar was such a helpful cleaning ingredient? Using glass containers and beeswax wraps to keep your food fresh and stored is a better alternative to plastic. It is also important to reuse bags, containers, and bottles multiple times as long as they are clean. Remember to check online for biodegradable products that are affordable and easily available near you. Once you change your products, you'll feel like your home is cleaner than before.

Moreover, your skin is your largest organ, and it is also the most susceptible to chemical reactions through toxic cosmetics. In addition to watching out for certain chemicals, here are a few ingredients that can be substituted. For example, hydroquinone can be substituted for Indian gooseberry or bearberry leaf for similar brightening effects, and synthetic fragrances can be replaced with natural scents such as cinnamon, rosemary, ginger, etc. Many healthy alternatives must be taken into consideration to live a safer lifestyle.

BECOMING YOUR OWN HEALTH ADVOCATE

We now know that menopause is not a taboo subject to be hidden from the world, especially from your doctor who can help you greatly in understanding your symptoms and recommend treatments according to your body's requirements.

Furthermore, many factors can cause menopausal symptoms to get worse or cause menopause to arrive earlier than usual. To understand all these things, it's best to have a professional's guidance while also doing your research.

First, make sure to do research and compile your concerns as questions before you meet your doctor. It is best to be prepared to grasp what they will be informing you about and to show your involvement with your health.

Second, it's important to be firm in understanding what they are saying and not be rushed into making decisions, but at the same time, be open to receiving advice. Make sure to clear any doubts and take your time with any decision regarding treatments.

Lastly, there are times when these appointments may seem too daunting, so if practicing your lines the day before or bringing emotional support helps you, take the steps you need to be comfortable.

There may be times when you don't agree with your doctor or aren't comfortable around them. In that case, it is best to find another doctor more suitable for you who can understand your point of view regarding your health. A capable doctor will do their utmost best to ease your worries.

The whole influx of new information, possible problems, and decisions that need to be taken responsibly can be a lot to take in. However, it's important to understand that everything must be taken into consideration with proper research to ensure that, even while in menopause, we can improve our lifestyle and minimize our struggles. Take these tips as a helping hand and look forward to a new burst of positivity.

7

MOVING FORWARD WITH
CONFIDENCE

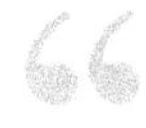

In this final chapter, we'll shift focus to connecting with your inner self during the unpredictable journey of menopause. This chapter will teach you all you need to know about embracing your postmenopausal life with grace. It will also guide you on how to find new interests, revamp your personal beauty, and learn to love yourself.

REBUILDING CONFIDENCE AFTER MENOPAUSE

As we know, menopause can bring out many physical and mental changes. It is common for women to feel a shift in their confidence levels as well. Unwanted weight gain, hormonal changes, and skincare problems can cause them to feel unworthy.

Rebuilding confidence after hitting menopause can be a tough challenge, but it's not impossible. You can take a holistic approach to all the changes you're going through.

The first step toward confidence has to be understanding. Once you educate yourself about menopause, its changes, myths, and misconceptions can help you create a strong foundation for understanding menopause and embracing it.

Let's discuss some easy-to-follow, time-tested strategies to embrace postmenopausal life:

- **Taking care of your mind and body:** It is vital to take care of yourself during the sometimes rough journey of menopause and life after. Self-care practices can enhance your confidence and well-being to a great extent. You can engage in activities such as daily walking, yoga, meditation, reading, or swimming. Not only will such activities improve your mood, but they will also balance your stress levels, making you more confident in how you look and feel. You should also try to eat a healthy and nutritious balanced diet. Giving yourself time to relax and do hobbies that you love can be empowering for your confidence. You'll feel relief during this transitional period and hone your self-esteem in the process.
- **Finding support networks:** At times, you may feel as if menopause is this harsh and lonely journey, where you might have no one to offer you their shoulder to lean on. However, it doesn't necessarily have to be this way. You can always connect with others who are also going through the same experiences and have a safe space to express yourself. A sense of belonging can provide the emotional support every woman needs. Join support groups that can provide you with great insight into your

menopausal symptoms. Once you start embracing menopause instead of treating it as something that weighs you down, you'll be able to navigate your way toward your confidence.

- **Seeking professional guidance:** Sometimes, you may feel as if the challenges and problems of menopause have overwhelmed you or have stressed you out. When this happens, you can opt for professional guidance. You can consult a healthcare professional who will help out with personalized advice and treatment options that will prove beneficial for you in the long run. They might also recommend therapy or other alternatives to ease your menopausal journey and boost your confidence.

- **Embracing changes:** Menopause is a journey that brings monumental changes to a woman's life. There is no denying that despite its tough nature, embracing changes positively can help you stay confident and strong. This change doesn't define a woman. Rather, it's just a phase that must be catered to carefully. To achieve that sense of confidence, it's important you redefine yourself through your own choices and not because of some societal norms. Set goals for yourself, try something new and exciting, and learn to live for yourself the way you want. This will provide a sense of achievement during menopause and beyond.

- **Boost your skin health:** For you to reach that ultimate level of confidence, it's important that you start taking care of the face you see all the time. Navigating your way to find out what skin products suit you best is indeed a tiring and time-consuming journey. However, it will prove to be fruitful if you find the right products and stick to a skincare regimen that will produce wonders for your skin. Stick to a healthy diet that has loads of fruits and vegetables that will keep your skin healthy and glowing as well.

Menopause brings many changes. Prioritizing yourself, nurturing your connections with others, and creating new hobbies can present you with the opportunity to grow and self-reflect. It allows you to envision your future the way you want, live in the moment as much as you can, and focus on what you need to make your life better. You can embark on a more purposeful journey and do things such as maintaining a journal, reconnecting with your old friends, or even learning a new language.

Contemplate your achievements, cherished memories, and the valuable lessons learned. With the wealth of experience gained through many successful years, postmenopausal life becomes a time to approach the future with newfound confidence and wisdom.

BEAUTY AND MENOPAUSE

As we know menopause brings many hormonal changes, especially the decline in the female hormone known as estrogen. These hormonal fluctuations can have a severe impact, especially on a woman's body. It also includes changes in the skin, hair, and overall appearance.

According to research, 42% of women claimed that amongst the changes that occurred in their menopausal transitional period, changes in their skin had to be the most distressing factor (*Skincare and the Menopause*, 2023).

So, let's enlighten you with some practical tips that you can opt for in your daily skincare routine according to your specific needs:

- **Hyaluronic acid:** To keep your skin healthy and plump, your dietary choices and skincare regimen have a concerning effect on your skin. If you don't have hyaluronic acid involved in your routine, then you are missing out on a crucial aspect. Hyaluronic acid has an exceptional ability to hold water. It can absorb and retain most of the water molecules and keep your skin hydrated. This is perfect for skin that is dry or dehydrated. As people age, the body's levels of hyaluronic acid fall. Hyaluronic acid can also aid in managing skin problems such as eczema. So, if you don't have this product in your routine, it's time you add it.

- **Sufficient sun protection:** If sunblock isn't a part of your routine, then you can end up with quite damaged skin and skin problems. Due to the harmful UV rays of the sun, protecting the skin becomes an imperative step. You must incorporate sunscreen into your skin routine to ensure that those harmful rays don't affect your skin. Always use a broad-spectrum sunscreen with at least SPF 30 or higher. Apply it all over your skin, especially on areas your clothing won't cover. Sunscreen helps your skin become spot-free, prevents new spots from forming, and significantly decreases your chance of getting skin cancer.

- **Dermatology support:** In recent years, pharmacy support has become a huge cause of help for women going through menopause and perimenopause.

Skin changes can be overwhelming, and women can lose their confidence when suffering from acne and other skin problems. Certain skin conditions can make your skin way more problematic than before, so pharmacists are in a good position to give women advice on this matter.

Pharmacists can give tips on how to take care of the skin and keep it hydrated. They might recommend using ingredients such as retinol and hyaluronic acid, which help support collagen production and strengthen the outer layer of the skin.

Hair Care Tips

Although you may feel envious of the hair commercials you see on the daily, they are a bit far-fetched and exaggerated. Those bouncy curls and voluminous hair may be your lifelong dream to achieve, and the truth is that you can attain that level of hair with the correct care and products.

Read through these hair-dos that are going to be a lifesaver, and turn your hair more healthy, shiny, and beautiful:

- **Wash your hair regularly:** You must ensure that you are washing your hair regularly, at least three days a week. It gets rid of the dirt and excess oil in the scalp. However, you must remember that the right frequency depends on the type of hair you have. For example, if you have an extremely dry scalp, try washing your hair only twice a week. If you have an oily scalp, then you can try washing your hair on alternate days. Remember to use lukewarm water for that shine on your hair. Super-hot water can strip your hair of its natural shine and make it appear dry and lifeless.
- **Use chemical-free shampoos:** You can't control what effect the environment has on your hair to a certain extent, but what you can do is not use shampoos that are loaded with chemicals. The less you use shampoos that are filled with every type of chemical, the healthier and prettier your hair will look. Choose the product that goes well with your

hair type, otherwise, you will end up damaging your hair one way or the other. Although sulfates and parabens are good for hair health, they can potentially cause skin irritation over time and disrupt your hormonal levels as well. Try to avoid products that contain those ingredients.

- **Condition correctly:** Your hair conditioner is responsible for making your hair fall straight and making it manageable. However, you must ensure that you apply the conditioner only to the tips of your hair and not the scalp. You should also be careful to rinse off all the product after applying it thoroughly. Remember, normal conditioner and leave-in conditioner are two different things.

- **Dry your hair naturally:** Excessive heat can damage your hair as well. Although blow drying can give your hair that pretty volume and make it look the same as movie stars and celebrities, it is not safe in the long run. You can use it to style your hair for important events, but ensure that you limit the use to certain times only. You can either air dry or towel dry. Don't use your towel harshly against the hair, as it can result in breakage. Remember to be gentle. Don't sleep with wet hair or comb your wet hair, as that too can result in breakage, damaged, and brittle hair.

- **Oil your hair properly:** Oiling your hair can increase your blood circulation to the scalp, relax your muscles, nourish the hair, and boost shine as well. Lather your hair generously with oil, focusing on the scalp and ends more. Oiling your hair can also retain your hair's moisture, enable your hair growth, and repair your split ends. Choose oils such as castor oil, olive oil, coconut oil, jojoba oil, almond oil, or any of your liking. Make sure you do this before you go to take a shower. You can leave the oil in for 20 minutes to two hours. Never sleep with your hair oiled, as that can clog your pores.

DISCOVERING NEW HOBBIES AND INTERESTS

Studies prove that having hobbies and interests can have a positive impact on your mental and physical health (*Finding Time for You*, 2023). Doing regular exercises, hanging out with friends, or even spending quality time alone can be exciting for you. Don't be afraid to get out of your comfort zone!

Let's look at the importance of hobbies and how they can change you for the better:

- **Reduce and manage stress:** I believe we can agree that menopause is quite a stressful time. New hobbies and interests can provide you with an effective way to get rid of, or at least manage, all that stress and anxiety that may come your way. Engaging in activities such as painting, reading, or even knitting can help you unwind and relax after a hectic day.
- **Challenge the brain, which can decrease cognitive decline:** Hobbies often require active engagement and problem-solving tactics, which then require continuous mental stimulation. This helps the brain keep active and supports the growth of new neural connections. It's also important to note that a nutritious diet, ample amount of exercise, and hobbies can contribute to maintaining a healthy brain that won't lose its cognitive abilities.
- **Support the immune system:** Problems like stress can suppress the immune system, making you more susceptible to diseases and conditions. Many hobbies help release endorphins, which are natural mood enhancers. This can help your immune system remain healthy accompanied with other healthy habits.

- **May support mobility:** We know that hobbies are mostly physical and can allow you to not only stay in good shape but also promote mobility. If you pick up hobbies such as martial arts, yoga, or meditation, these can improve your balance and coordination, which in turn can help you prevent falling. Strength training can also aid in improving your joints and gaining muscle mass that would aid in eliminating body fat.
- **May improve social connections that can enhance one's mood:** Joining group activities or playing team sports is not only about making friends; it also helps you stay active. Being around others can motivate you to keep moving and make exercise more enjoyable.

Whether your hobby is cooking or gardening, writing or traveling, or you're trying something new, you'll never be bored or wonder how to fill your day. This will help you stay active and happy as well.

Once you start sticking to hobbies that make you satisfied, relaxed, and mellow, it will result in you handling your menopause journey way better than you had thought. You can opt for hobbies such as arts and crafts, cooking, baking, making jewelry, sports, and so many other options you can avail.

If you are someone who gets bored of just sitting around, you can also travel or listen to your favorite music while you work. Board games and journaling may also be a great idea to get you started on hobbies.

EMBRACING THE NEW YOU

Embracing and loving yourself through all the stages of menopause is what is going to help you push through the challenges and hardships with confidence and ease. Acceptance helps us foster a positive mindset, aids us in navigating through problems, and gives us a graceful outlook on life.

The acceptance of new changes in your body, mind, and overall self is what's going to promote mental and emotional resilience, contributing to a more fulfilling and joyful postmenopause experience.

Remember to be kind and compassionate to yourself even on days you don't feel like the best version of yourself. You get to decide what wellness and happiness mean to you and form your days according to that. Don't subscribe to other people's definition of fun. Do what is best for you and know that you are not being selfish about it.

Don't fear menopause or think of it as a mark on your life where everything is going to go downhill. It's never been like that, and it's not going to be. Read aloud positive affirmations while looking yourself in the mirror and let a positive mindset process life for you.

You have no reason to stop living life the way it is or hate yourself for the natural change that occurred within you. Tell yourself that you are beautiful no matter what and that you'll treat menopause like a change that will alter you too for the better.

You'd have the opportunity to be yourself, not have to worry about periods and pregnancy, and, best of all, not let your mood swings take the best of you. Say goodbye to those awful cramps forever!

WORKING TOWARD LONGEVITY

The idea that the secrets of longevity are hidden in the ovaries refers to the potential role of certain hormones and cellular processes associated with the female reproductive system in influencing the overall life span.

As menopause causes female hormones such as estrogen and progesterone to decline, bone density decreases, the risk of fractures increases, and stroke and other problems become more inevitable. All these factors jeopardize our long-term health, and menopausal symptoms can decrease our longevity.

While the ovaries and hormones may play a role in certain aspects of living a longer life, it's crucial to recognize that factors such as genetics, lifestyle decisions, and environmental influences also have substantial impacts on determining how long a person lives.

To enhance your longevity, you can exercise well, eat healthily, quit smoking, reduce stress levels by finding good hobbies, wear layered clothes as per your feeling hot or cold, maintain social connections, alleviate your mental health, get hormone replacement therapy, shield your immune system, and treat menopause like a natural transition in your life, not a disease.

After a full year without menstruation, you enter the post-menopausal stage, a positive phase of life. Should you notice any postmenopausal bleeding, inform your doctor promptly, as this is not typical and requires further evaluation. If you encounter persistent issues related to sleep, focus, mood, hot flashes, urinary function, or reduced libido, it's advisable to discuss them with your physician, as there may be other underlying conditions that need attention.

Menopause is a reality that becomes a catalyst for positive trans-formation, setting the stage for a vibrant and fulfilling life ahead. Believe that you can become the best version of yourself while staying comfortable and being confident throughout.

We have explored the transformative journey of menopause, emphasizing ideas such as embracing changes, discovering new sources of joy, and moving forward with utmost confidence. The idea is that menopause is not the endpoint but a pivotal gateway to a new chapter of life. It's an opportunity for women to redefine their identities while seeking and celebrating new moments of joy.

In conclusion, it's vital that we as women pull each other up and give space to become the best versions of ourselves. Treat menopause as a gateway to new adventures that await us all!

Empowering Other Women

Now you have everything you need to CONQUER MENOPAUSE, it's time to pass on your newfound knowledge and show other readers where they can find the same help. Would you extend a helping hand to someone you've never met, even without expecting credit for it? Whether it's a friend, a family member, or a stranger seeking guidance, your words could make all the difference. Your gift doesn't cost a dime and takes less than 60 seconds to give, but it can change a fellow reader's life forever. Your review could help...

...a woman find solace in her journey.
...a caregiver better support their loved one.
...a community foster open and honest conversations.
...a reader discover the strength within themselves.
...a ripple effect of positivity and empowerment.

To make a real difference and experience that 'feel-good' moment, all you have to do is leave a review. Scan the QR code below to share your thoughts:

Thank you for being part of this journey and for your commitment to empowering others. Together, we can keep the game of conquering menopause alive and thriving.

Warmest regards,

Samarra James

CONCLUSION

We began this book eager to learn more about menopause and its impact on our lives with perhaps no idea where to begin. Every page brought us new information, and even if we were scared of the negative sides of menopause and the pain that can come with it, we learned how to navigate through this important phase in a woman's life and how to adapt to the changes it brings—good and bad.

Embarking on this journey, even if we come in different shapes, ages, and walks of life, we are now equipped with the knowledge we need to prepare and adapt to the menopause stage. Moreover, we can gain the courage to realize that we are not alone in this experience and that every reader of this book can relate to its message. You have a support group right before your eyes. We may have started with little to no clue about menopause, but I'd like to say that now, we've learned a great deal. That being said, here are a few things to remember:

Know that you are more than a woman who is experiencing the "end" of your youth. You aren't an over dramatic or emotional mess, nor are your feelings and concerns to be pushed aside for the sake of not being a burden to others. You are a powerful being capable of growth, learning, and adapting to situations even when the world seems to be against you.

Menopause and the pain that can come with it, such as headaches, hot flashes, etc., can be scary. However, now equipped with the knowledge of this book, you have multiple doors open to you. The only thing to do now is to make the correct decisions and choose the correct doors for you. The correct decisions shouldn't only be actions that you must take to make your menopause easier on yourself, but also for those around you to offer support and love during this time. Never downplay your suffering; remember to talk to others because communication is key for your peace of mind and for others to understand you. Most importantly, this communication will improve your relationship with your family and partner. We can forget the stats of divorcing women at the age of their menopause and focus on a healthy relationship together.

Spread your newly gained knowledge to others who either are or will be susceptible to experiencing menopause as well. Create a powerful and protective community so you can stand together even when no one stands with you. Never stop learning about your body and find new ways to love yourself in your purest form. You are more powerful than what you perceive yourself to be. Take each day at a time and learn to value the person you see in the mirror.

Menopause shouldn't restrain you from being active or productive. With safe ways to reduce menopausal symptoms, you can continue a healthy and productive lifestyle with vigor and energy. Of course, it's important not to push yourself too hard and take ample rest as well. Focus on yourself and enjoy your off days to the fullest by doing the most mundane things if it brings you joy.

It is understandable that the influx of information about something we never realized the importance of makes us feel as if we have been missing out on something all our lives. That is where the responsibility of learning comes in. Research about your body and the things happening in it to be more aware and concerned about your health. Take interest in what the doctor suggests and initiate conversations with them to make sure you are getting your point across while respecting their expertise with confidence.

I will implore you to never lose that curiosity or drive that helped you pick this book to learn and understand. We will always go through many phases in our lives; however, with knowledge regarding it, we can be prepared and welcome the change with open arms and an open mind. Menopause may be a battle, but armed with this book, you are sure to claim victory by the end of it.

REFERENCES

Ayres, N. (2022, October 14). *How to cope with menopause symptoms at work*. Prime Health. https://www.prime-health.co.uk/blog/how-to-cope-with-menopause-symptoms-at-work

Best supplements for menopause. (2022, October 26). Cleveland Clinic Health Essentials. https://health.clevelandclinic.org/menopause-supplements

Brennan, D. (2021, September 27). *Intermittent fasting for women over 50: What you need to know*. WebMD. https://www.webmd.com/healthy-aging/what-to-know-about-intermittent-fasting-for-women-after-50

Breaking down barriers to fitness. (2018, April 18). American Heart Association. https://www.heart.org/en/healthy-living/fitness/getting-active/breaking-down-barriers-to-fitness

Britto, J. (2021, October 1). *How do you bounce back sexually after menopause?* Healthline. https://www.healthline.com/health/healthy-sex/how-do-you-bounce-back-sexually-after-menopause#1

Brown, M. J.. (2023, April 21). *11 natural remedies for menopause relief*. Healthline. https://www.healthline.com/nutrition/11-natural-menopause-tips

Bygraves, M., & Witton, N. (2021, August 3). *7 relaxation techniques for sleep that actually work*. Kokoon. https://kokoon.io/blogs/bufferzone/relaxation-techniques-for-sleep

Can you change your circadian Rhythm? (2024, January 3). Sleep Foundation. https://www.sleepfoundation.org/circadian-rhythm/can-you-change-your-circadian-rhythm

Caring for your skin in menopause. (2023, November 20). American Academy of Dermatology. https://www.aad.org/public/everyday-care/skin-care-secrets/anti-aging/skin-care-during-menopause

Changes in hormone levels, sexual side effects of menopause. (n.d.). North American Menopause Society. https://www.menopause.org/for-women/sexual-health-menopause-online/changes-at-midlife/changes-in-hormone-levels

Charity, M. (2021, October 21). *How to ask your GP for help*. The Menopause Charity. https://www.themenopausecharity.org/2021/10/21/how-to-ask-your-gp-for-help

Chemicals in the home. (n.d.). Better Health Channel. https://www.betterhealth.vic.gov.au/health/healthyliving/Chemicals-in-the-home

Chemical safety in the home. (2024, January 15). Nidirect. https://www.nidirect.gov.uk/articles/chemical-safety-home#:~:

Cloyd, K. (2023, October 10). *Using the Gut Zoomer test in clinic.* Rupa Health. https://www.rupahealth.com/post/using-the-gut-zoomer-test-in-clinic

Cohen, M. (2022, July 26). *7 best exercises for menopause symptoms, including weight gain.* Good Housekeeping. https://www.goodhousekeeping.com/health/fitness/g40476189/menopause-exercises

Coppa, A. M. (n.d.). *10 tips to managing your menopause symptoms at work.* A. Michael Coppa, M.D. https://www.drcoppaobgyn.com/blog/10-tips-to-managing-your-menopause-symptoms-at-work

Dasgupta, R. (2020, August 17). *Sleep hygiene explained and 10 tips for better sleep.* Healthline. https://www.healthline.com/health/sleep-hygiene#bed-and-sleep

DePolo, J. (n.d.). *Post-menopausal health concerns and how to manage them.* Breastcancer.org. https://www.breastcancer.org/treatment-side-effects/menopause/postmenopause

Discovering menopause relief with infrared sauna therapy. (2023, September 18). Sunlighten. https://www.sunlighten.com/gb-en/blog/menopause-relief-with-infrared-sauna-therapy

Dolgen, E. (2017, December 7). *How to maintain a healthy relationship, even during menopause.* HuffPost. https://www.huffpost.com/entry/how-to-maintain-a-healthy_b_6045508

Donsky, A. (2022, July 21). *Family support during menopause.* Morphus. https://wearemorphus.com/blogs/relationships/family-support-during-menopause

Don't sweat it: Busting six menopause myths. (2022, March 22). UVM Health Network. https://www.uvmhealth.org/healthsource/dont-sweat-it-busting-six-menopause-myths

Dressing through and beyond the menopause. (2022, July 31). Image Consultant & Personal Stylist. https://www.kerrieellis.co.uk/2022/07/31/dressing-through-and-beyond-the-menopause/

Dunne, L. (2022, May 10). *How to talk to your manager about menopause.* Health & Her. https://healthandher.com/hot-topics/how-to-talk-to-your-manager-about-menopause

Earlier menopause linked to everyday chemical exposures. (2015, January 15). ScienceDaily. https://www.sciencedaily.com/releases/2015/01/150128141417.htm#:~:

Easy ways to boost self-confidence during menopause. (2021, April 8). Emepelle. https://emepelle.co.uk/blogs/emepelle-edit/easy-ways-to-boost-self-confidence-during-menopause

Effective stress management techniques during Menopause. (2023, August 8). Vitali-Natura Essentials. https://www.vitalinatura.com/blogs/dailydose/effective-stress-management-techniques-for-women-during-menopause

Eiser, S. E. (2021, September 23). *Is Menopause keeping you awake?* Lancaster General Health. https://www.lancastergeneralhealth.org/health-hub-home/2021/september/is-menopause-keeping-you-awake-tips-for-getting-a-good-nights-sleep

Feller, D. (2023, November 3). *Birth control and menopause: At what age should you stop taking birth control pills?* HealthPartners Blog. https://www.healthpartners.com/blog/birth-control-and-menopause/#

Fernandes, R. (2023, March 28). *Understanding Menopause: A Natural Biological Process in a Woman's Life.* Supplement Hub. https://supplementhub.com/blog/menopause

Finding time for you. (2023, May 3). The Menopause Charity. https://www.themenopausecharity.org/2023/05/03/finding-time-for-you

Five menopause myths you should stop believing now. (2023, February 7). NYU Langone Health. https://nyulangone.org/news/five-menopause-myths-you-should-stop-believing-now

5 reasons to walk more during menopause. (2023, April 24). Balance Menopause. https://www.balance-menopause.com/menopause-library/5-reasons-to-walk-more-during-the-menopause

Foster, J. (2022, February 25). *What going through menopause at the same time your partner is like.* Yahoo. https://uk.style.yahoo.com/lgbt-month-same-sex-couple-double-menopause-152610730.html?guccounter=1&guce_referrer=aHR0cH M6Ly93d3cuZ29vZ2xlLmNvbS8&guce_referrer_sig=AQAAAJGFoekUF f54PH7xwYC84N3ysiFBHlF-AS9_-MqLs6Y6yCSHma1QoUDfn3gEIpupO-rnJB8eyVA8m67WVKRYOnqO5-DYmuzu7RX0mj_y07_d2WajtedwmCZ52-36nXyQpqqXAjughN1p2TUmhVxrm0Um_6b16abhGAwp6U6a_QcB

Garcia, J. (2023, October 19). *Red light therapy for menopause.* Infraredi. https://infraredi.asia/blogs/red-light-therapy/red-light-therapy-for-menopause

Gordon, D. (2021, July 13). *73% of Women Don't Treat Their Menopause Symptoms, New Survey Shows.* Forbes. https://www.forbes.com/sites/debgordon/2021/07/13/73-of-women-dont-treat-their-menopause-symptoms-new-survey-shows/?sh=4ae6df71454f

Grey, H. (2022, October 4). *Talking with Your Doctor About Menopause: Where Do I Even Start?* Healthline. https://www.healthline.com/health/menopause/talking-with-your-doctor

A guide to embracing menopause. (2023, March 16). Surya Prana Nutrition. https://www.suryaprananutrition.co.uk/blog/a-guide-to-embracing-menopause

Having "the talk": Top tips for discussing your menopause with loved ones. Holland & Barrett. (2023, August 21). https://www.hollandandbarrett.com/the-health-hub/conditions/womens-health/menopause/talk-about-menopause

Hormone therapy for menopause symptoms. (n.d.). Cleveland Clinic. https://my.cleve

landclinic.org/health/treatments/15245-hormone-therapy-for-menopause-symptoms

How can I talk to my family and friends about my menopause symptoms? (n.d.). StoryMD. https://storymd.com/journal/m9kx4yrtgw-menopause-symptoms/page/or826hv5el3-how-can-i-talk-to-my-family-and-friends-about-my-menopause-symptoms

How can menopause affect sleep? (2022, December 15). Sleep Foundation. https://www.sleepfoundation.org/women-sleep/menopause-and-sleep

How to make a sleep-friendly bedroom. (2020, November 10). National Sleep Foundation. https://www.thensf.org/how-to-make-a-sleep-friendly-bedroom

How to talk to your family about menopause. (2023, December 21). My Menopause Centre. https://www.mymenopausecentre.com/blog/how-to-talk-about-the-menopause

How to boost confidence in menopause. (2023, September 27). The Menopause Charity. https://www.themenopausecharity.org/2023/09/27/boost-confidence

It's not all bad: 5 positive parts of menopause. (n.d.). A. Michael Coppa, M.D. https://www.drcoppaobgyn.com/blog/its-not-all-bad-5-positive-parts-of-menopause

Jacobs, D. (2023, October 13). *How to strengthen romantic relationships in menopause.* MenoLabs. https://menolabs.com/blogs/menolife/how-to-strengthen-romantic-relationships-in-menopause

Jaliman, D. (2023, February 25). *Slideshow: 19 hair care tips.* WebMD. https://www.webmd.com/beauty/ss/slideshow-best-kept-hair-secrets

Johnson, T. C. (2022, August 11). *Menopause diet/foods: What to eat & what to avoid.* WebMD. https://www.webmd.com/menopause/staying-healthy-through-good-nuitrition

Johnson, T. C. (2022, November 20). *11 supplements for menopause symptoms.* WebMD. https://www.webmd.com/menopause/ss/slideshow-menopause

Jones, J. (2022, January 18). *Keto and menopause: Is it a good diet for hormones?* Medical News Today. https://www.medicalnewstoday.com/articles/keto-and-menopause#keto-diet

Kristen. (2023b, October 20). *Eco-friendly alternatives to common household products.* Earth Friendly Tips. https://earthfriendlytips.com/eco-friendly-alternatives-to-common-products

Kubala, J. (2018, June 28). *The 9 best keto supplements.* Healthline. https://www.healthline.com/nutrition/best-keto-supplements#TOC_TITLE_HDR_4

Levine, B., & Smythe, K. L. (n.d.). *10 symptoms of menopause and perimenopause.* Everyday Health. https://www.everydayhealth.com/menopause/perimenopause-symptoms

Learning about healthy eating during menopause. (n.d.). My Health Alberta. https://

myhealth.alberta.ca/Health/aftercareinformation/pages/conditions.aspx?hwid=abk7408

Learning to love menopause. (2020, December 2). Chester County Hospital. https://www.chestercountyhospital.org/news/health-eliving-blog/2020/december/learning-to-love-menopause

Levine, B., & Smythe, K. L. (n.d.). *10 symptoms of menopause and perimenopause.* Everyday Health. https://www.everydayhealth.com/menopause/perimenopause-symptoms

Lopez, I. (2021, September 23). *Are harmful chemicals hiding in your cosmetics?* WebMD. https://www.webmd.com/beauty/features/harmful-chemicals-in-your-cosmetics

Make time for exercise with these 9 simple tips. (2019, June 18). Polar. https://www.polar.com/blog/9-ways-how-to-make-time-for-exercise

Managing work-life balance during menopause. (2022, June 12). Woombie. https://woombie.com/blog/post/managing-work-life-balance-during-menopause

Manning, M. (2023, July 9). *Hobbies for women over 50.* Sixty and Me. https://sixtyandme.com/list-of-hobbies-for-women-over-50

Menopause. (2022, October 17). World Health Organization. https://www.who.int/news-room/fact-sheets/detail/menopause

Menopause and longevity. (n.d.). Femgevity Health. https://www.femgevityhealth.com/blog/aging-with-intention-using-menopause-to-improve-your-longevity

Menopause and the workplace. (2023, January 31). NHS Inform. https://www.nhsinform.scot/healthy-living/womens-health/later-years-around-50-years-and-over/menopause-and-post-menopause-health/menopause-and-the-workplace

Menopause and your mental wellbeing. (2022, November 29). NHS inform. https://www.nhsinform.scot/healthy-living/womens-health/later-years-around-50-years-and-over/menopause-and-post-menopause-health/menopause-and-your-mental-wellbeing

Menopause as a time of new beginnings. (n.d.). North American Menopause Society. https://www.menopause.org/for-women/sexual-health-menopause-online/reminders-and-resources/menopause-as-a-time-of-new-beginnings

Menopause and weight. (n.d.). Better Health Channel. https://www.betterhealth.vic.gov.au/health/conditionsandtreatments/menopause-and-weight-gain

Menopause - Diagnosis and treatment (2017). Mayo Clinic. https://www.mayoclinic.org/diseases-conditions/menopause/diagnosis-treatment/drc-20353401

Menopause in the workplace – How to improve your experience. (2022, August 26). The Marion Gluck Clinic. https://www.mariongluckclinic.com/blog/menopause-in-the-workplace-practical-tips-for-improving-your-experience-at-work.html

Menopause hormone therapy (HT) benefits & risks. The North American Menopause

Society. (n.d.). https://www.menopause.org/for-women/menopauseflashes/menopause-symptoms-and-treatments/hormone-therapy-benefits-risks

Migala, J., & Anderson, K. (2023, July 24). *12 low-carb diets: Keto, low-carb paleo, Atkins, and more.* Everyday Health. https://www.everydayhealth.com/diet-nutrition/diet/low-carb-diets-keto-low-carb-paleo-atkins-more

Migala, J., & Laube, J. (2022, November 22). *What is tai chi? A guide to tai chi for beginners.* Everyday Health. https://www.everydayhealth.com/wellness/tai-chi/guide

Myers, W., & Laube, J. (2023, April 28). *8 ways to sit less and move more each day.* Everyday Health. https://www.everydayhealth.com/fitness/neat-exercises-for-couch-potatoes.aspx

My story: How regular exercise helped me manage my menopause symptoms. (2023, November 28). BOMIMO. https://bomimonutrition.com/blogs/news/how-regular-exercise-menopause-symptoms

Munn, C., Vaughan, L., Talaulikar, V., Davies, M. C., & Harper, J. C. (2022). Menopause knowledge and education in women under 40: Results from an online survey. *Women's Health.* https://doi.org/10.1177/17455057221139660

Nalwoga, B. (n.d.). *Bad keto fats: Which ones to avoid & what to eat instead.* Perfect Keto. https://perfectketo.com/bad-keto-fats

Natural treatments for menopause Symptoms. (2006, December 31). WebMD. https://www.webmd.com/menopause/menopause-natural-treatments

Neumann, K. D. (2023, August 17). *What is biohacking and how does it work? Forbes Health.* https://www.forbes.com/health/wellness/biohacking/#:~:text=Bio-hacking%20is%20the%20practice%20of,Lofton%2C%20a%20registered%20di-etitian%20and

9 ways to manage stress and relax during menopause. (n.d.). Australian Menopause Centre. https://www.menopausecentre.com.au/information-centre/articles/9-ways-to-manage-stress-and-relax-during-menopause

9 yogic breathing practices for mind-body balance and healing. (n.d.). https://www.himalayanyogainstitute.com/9-yogic-breathing-practices-mind-body-balance-healing/

No time for exercise? Here are 7 easy ways to move more! (2017, December 13). American Heart Association. https://www.heart.org/en/healthy-living/fitness/getting-active/no-time-for-exercise-here-are-7-easy-ways-to-move-more

Oakley, K. (n.d.). *The best exercise routines during menopause.* Stella. https://www.onstella.com/the-latest/long-term-health/the-best-exercise-for-menopause/

O'Neill, M., Jones, V. F., & Reid, A. (2023). *Impact of menopausal symptoms on work and careers: a cross-sectional study. Occupational Medicine, 73*(6), 332–338. https://doi.org/10.1093/occmed/kqad078

Palladino, A., & Brown, M. J. (2018, November 23). *Menopause diet: How what you eat affects your symptoms.* Healthline. https://www.healthline.com/nutrition/menopause-diet#foods-to-eat

Payne, J. M. (2021, February 18). *Why you should exercise your way through menopause.* Lancaster General Health. https://www.lancastergeneralhealth.org/health-hub-home/2021/february/why-you-should-exercise-your-way-through-menopause

Perimenopause - Symptoms and causes. (2023, May 25). Mayo Clinic. https://www.mayoclinic.org/diseases-conditions/perimenopause/symptoms-causes/syc-20354666

Pien, G. W. (n.d.). *How does menopause affect my sleep?* Johns Hopkins Medicine. https://www.hopkinsmedicine.org/health/wellness-and-prevention/how-does-menopause-affect-my-sleep

Pierson, C. (2022, October 26). *How infrared saunas help to balance hormones and improve menstrual cramps and menopausal symptoms.* The Float Spa. https://www.thefloatspa.co.uk/how-infrared-saunas-help-to-balance-hormones-and-improve-menstrual-cramps-and-menopausal-symptoms/#:~:

PEMF Therapy for Menopause. (2021, October 5). PEMP Devices. https://www.pemf-devices.com/menopause-pemf/

Perry, S., & Linville, K. (n.d.). *Menopause and dehydration: Drink more water.* Gennev. https://www.gennev.com/education/menopause-and-dehydration

Postmenopause: Signs, symptoms, & treatments. (n.d.). University of Utah Health. https://healthcare.utah.edu/womens-health/gynecology/menopause/postmenopause

Relaxation exercises to help fall asleep. (2023, December 22). Sleep Foundation. https://www.sleepfoundation.org/sleep-hygiene/relaxation-exercises-to-help-fall-asleep

Safe alternatives for 8 toxic skincare ingredients. (2017, April 19). American Spa. https://www.americanspa.com/skincare/safe-alternatives-8-toxic-skincare-ingredients

Satmary, W. A., & Dresden, D. (2021, December 23). *Do menopause supplements work?* Medical News Today. https://www.medicalnewstoday.com/articles/menopause-supplements#calcium-and-vitamin-d

Scerbo, B. (2023, June 29). *How to celebrate your body during menopause.* The Change is Personal. https://thechangeispersonal.com/mastering-menopause/how-to-celebrate-your-body-during-menopause-a-body-positive-approach/

Schmidt C. W. (2017). *Age at menopause: Do chemical exposures play a role? Environmental health perspectives, 125*(6), 062001. https://doi.org/10.1289/EHP2093

7 menopausal benefits of a 10-minute walk. (2019, December 23). A.Vogel. https://www.avogel.co.uk/health/menopause/videos/7-menopausal-benefits-of-a-10-minute-walk/

Sex and menopause. (n.d.). Menopause. https://www.menopause.org/for-women/

menopauseflashes/sexual-health/how-to-increase-your-sexual-desire-during-menopause#

Singh, A., & Varma, A. (2023). *Whole-body vibration therapy as a modality for treatment of senile and postmenopausal osteoporosis.* Cureus. https://doi.org/10.7759/cureus.33690

Simmonds, L. (2022, January 23). *Style tips for menopausal women.* The Fearless Fashionista. https://thefearlessfashionista.com/blog/style-tips-4-menopausal-women-2zdhx

6 expert tips for setting realistic fitness goals. (2023, October 31). Forbes. https://www.forbes.com/health/fitness/setting-realistic-fitness-goals

6 ways to find relief from your menopause symptoms. (2023, December 18). Cleveland Clinic. https://health.clevelandclinic.org/natural-menopause-remedies

Sleep apnea - Symptoms and causes. (2023, April 6). Mayo Clinic. https://www.mayoclinic.org/diseases-conditions/sleep-apnea/symptoms-causes/syc-20377631

Sleep problems and menopause: What can I do? (2021, September 30). National Institute on Aging. https://www.nia.nih.gov/health/menopause/sleep-problems-and-menopause-what-can-i-do

Skincare and the menopause. (2023, September 13). Pharmacy Magazine. https://www.pharmacymagazine.co.uk/clinical/skincare-and-the-menopause

Sreenivas, S. (2021, May 3). *Birth control during menopause.* WebMD. https://www.webmd.com/sex/birth-control/birth-control-during-menopause

Stanten, M., & Linville, K. (2021, September 14). *Get moving in menopause: 50 benefits of walking.* Gennev. https://www.gennev.com/education/benefits-walking-menopause

Talking about menopause with friends and family. (n.d.). Australian Menopause Centre. https://www.menopausecentre.com.au/information-centre/articles/talking-about-menopause-with-friends-and-family

Talking to your doctor about the menopause. (2024, January 4). Theramex. https://www.theramex.com/talking-to-your-doctor-about-the-menopause

Tamatam, S. (2022, January 17). *Top hair care tips straight from the experts.* SkinKraft. https://skinkraft.com/blogs/articles/hair-care-tips

10 steps to avoid toxic chemicals. (2020, January 9). Women's Voices for the Earth. https://womensvoices.org/avoid-toxic-chemicals/ten-ways-to-avoid-toxic-chemicals

Top 5 reasons you should be using the DUTCH test. (n.d.). Golden Leaf Health Center. https://goldenleafhc.com/top-5-reasons-you-should-be-using-the-dutch-test

The reality of menopause weight gain. (2023, July 8). Mayo Clinic. https://www.mayoclinic.org/healthy-lifestyle/womens-health/in-depth/menopause-weight-gain/art-20046058

The water in you: Water and the human body. (n.d.). USGS. https://www.usgs.gov/special-topics/water-science-school/science/water-you-water-and-human-body

The benefits of exercise during menopause. (2015, April 28). Australian Menopause Centre. https://www.menopausecentre.com.au/information-centre/articles/the-benefits-of-exercise-during-menopause

30 fun ways to exercise. (n.d.). Cancer Research UK. https://www.cancerresearchuk.org/get-involved/find-an-event/the-exercise-challenge/30-ways-to-exercise

The health benefits of social support during the menopausal transition. (n.d.). Menopause Natural Solutions. https://www.menopausenaturalsolutions.com/blog/social-support

The 34 symptoms of menopause, PEMF therapy helps. (2021, March 6). Centurion Tesla Technology for Health. https://www.centurion-systems.com/the-34-symptoms-of-the-menopause-pemf-therapy-helps

The use of neurofeedback in dealing with menopause. (n.d.). BEE Medic. https://beemedic.com/en/use-neurofeedback-dealing-menopause-0

Upham, B., & Smythe, K. L. (2023, May 23). *10 reasons to look forward to menopause.* Everyday Health. https://www.everydayhealth.com/menopause-pictures/positives-of-menopause.aspx

Upham, B., & Franco, R. (2023, June 14). *Healthy foods for menopause.* Everyday Health. https://www.everydayhealth.com/menopause/healthy-foods-to-eat-during-menopause/

Urbanski, B. (2022b, October 18). *Menopause puts final nail in marriage coffin.* Balance Menopause. https://www.balance-menopause.com/news/menopause-puts-final-nail-in-marriage-coffin/

Vargo, B. (n.d.). *Deep breathing and relaxation in yoga.* Arthritis Foundation. https://www.arthritis.org/health-wellness/healthy-living/physical-activity/yoga/deep-breathing-and-relaxation-in-yoga

Vermaak, C. (n.d.). *Barriers to physical activity.* Physiopedia. https://www.physiopedia.com/Barriers_to_Physical_Activity

Ways to self-advocate at your doctor's appointment. (n.d.). Banner Health. https://www.bannerhealth.com/healthcareblog/advise-me/advocating-for-yourself-when-youre-talking-to-your-doctor

We are what we eat. (n.d.). NCBI. https://www.ncbi.nlm.nih.gov/pmc/articles/PMC9616445/

Werner, C. (2023, September 7). *10 tips for how to advocate for yourself at the doctor.* Healthline. https://www.healthline.com/health/how-to-advocate-for-yourself-at-the-doctor

West, H. (2017, June 3). *20 clever tips to eat healthy when eating out.* Healthline.

https://www.healthline.com/nutrition/20-healthy-tips-for-eating-out#TOC_TITLE_HDR_17

Wetmore, K. (2023, February 8). *Hormone replacement therapy: Is it right for you?* (n.d.). Cedars-Sinai. https://www.cedars-sinai.org/blog/hormone-replacement-therapy-risks-benefits.html

What are the benefits of red light therapy? (n.d.). Rouge Care. https://global.rougecare.ca/pages/what-are-the-benefits-of-red-light-therapy?shpxid=73bc2f79-c975-4ae8-a3b7-3e21b24b8981

Which hormones affect sleep? 5 hormones to know about. (2022, March 9). Sleep Centers of Middle Tennessee. https://sleepcenterinfo.com/blog/which-hormones-affect-sleep

WHN Editorial Team. (2022, January 19). *Rekindling desire — the soul of your libido.* Women's Health Network. https://www.womenshealthnetwork.com/menopause-and-perimenopause/rekindling-desire-rebuilding-libido

Wild, S. (2023, February 1). *What's the best exercise for the menopause?* Bupa UK. https://www.bupa.co.uk/newsroom/ourviews/menopause-exercise

Glamour. (2023, October 9). 13 Celebrities Who Have Spoken Out About Menopause. Glamour. Retrieved April 28, 2024, from https://www.glamour.com/gallery/celebrities-who-have-spoken-out-about-menopause